LYSOS●MAL STORAGE DIS●RDERS

Principles and Practice

LYSOS●MAL STORAGE DIS●RDERS

Principles and Practice

Gregory M. Pastores

New York University School of Medicine, USA

World Scientific

NEW JERSEY · LONDON · SINGAPORE · BEIJING · SHANGHAI · HONG KONG · TAIPEI · CHENNAI

Published by

World Scientific Publishing Co. Pte. Ltd.

5 Toh Tuck Link, Singapore 596224

USA office: 27 Warren Street, Suite 401-402, Hackensack, NJ 07601

UK office: 57 Shelton Street, Covent Garden, London WC2H 9HE

British Library Cataloguing-in-Publication Data
A catalogue record for this book is available from the British Library.

LYSOSOMAL STORAGE DISORDERS
Principles and Practice

ISBN-13 978-981-4271-31-8
ISBN-10 981-4271-31-4

Typeset by Stallion Press
Email: enquiries@stallionpress.com

Foreword

Over the past few decades we have seen remarkable progress in our understanding of the lysosomal storage diseases (LSDs) thanks to many physicians and scientists who have devoted their careers to unraveling the clinical, biochemical and molecular intricacies of these rare disorders. Dr Pastores has been both a witness and a contributor to the emergence of this field close to the forefront of medical genetics. This concise guide is a distillation of his experiences caring for patients, teaching medical students, residents and fellows, conducting clinical trials and participation in national and international meetings devoted to progress in the LSDs.

He begins by emphasizing that these disorders involve all age groups and multiple organ systems so that physicians caring for both children and adults and from all specialties need to be informed. Historical information of each disorder and vignettes liven up the text. The complexity of diagnosis is simplified by an emphasis on clinical signs and a paradigm for diagnostic testing. Guidance is given on biochemical and molecular testing and prenatal diagnosis and screening for carriers. Laboratory pitfalls such as pseudo-deficiency alleles and activator protein deficiencies are addressed in this well-referenced and up-to-date monograph. Disease mechanisms, a relatively new field of inquiry, are nicely summarized yet there is much about pathogenesis of the LSDs that remains unknown. However, what makes the LSDs of such great interest today are the multiple approaches to therapy, some already in use and others in clinical trials and potentially promising. To measure treatment progress, disease-specific scoring systems are needed as well as quality of life measures and these are also well-covered. The many tables in this manual allow even the beginning student convenient shortcuts to differentiate the various LSDs on clinical grounds.

Even though rare, the LSDs continue to spawn new insights into basic molecular processes with the potential for wider applications to other categories of genetic disease. Both new and established students of the LSDs will find this book a roadmap not only for better case finding and management but also a stimulus to continue the tradition of discovery that is the lifeblood of academic medicine.

Edwin H. Kolodny, M.D.
Bernard A. and Charlotte Marden Professor of Neurology
Chairman, Department of Neurology
New York University School of Medicine
New York, USA

Preface

*We ought not to set them aside with idle thoughts or idle words about
'curiosities' or 'chances'. Not one of them is without meaning; not one
that might not become the beginning of excellent knowledge, if only we
could answer the question — why is it rare or being rare, why did it in
this instance happen?*

— James Paget (1882)

I had the good fortune of coming to Mount Sinai Medical Center
(MSMC), New York to complete my training in medical genetics, after
an initial period of grounding at the Mayo Clinic in Minnesota. At that
time (1990), enzyme therapy for Gaucher disease (GD) was in clinical
trials. As New York had a large Ashkenazi Jewish community and GD
was a prevalent and well-characterized disorder in this population,
patient recruitment would not be a problem. Furthermore, a physician at
MSMC (Gregory A. Grabowski) had up to that point devoted most of
his professional life to studying the disease. Thus, our group had anticipated being involved in the pivotal trials to evaluate the recombinant
form of glucocerebrosidase (the enzyme deficient in GD). When Greg
left for Ohio in 1991 to head the Division of Genetics at the Children's
Hospital in Cincinnati, I took over the care of our GD patients and com-
pletion of the trials, which was then a collaborative effort between
MSMC and Norman Barton and Roscoe O. Brady at the National
Institutes of Health. Roscoe's role was both vital and of special interest,

as he had in the mid-60's delineated the enzyme deficiency that was shown to cause GD and proposed the feasibility of treatment by infusing the protein, isolated from human placenta, into patients. These initiatives were supported by Genzyme Corporation, and facilitated by Orphan Drug legislation (established in 1983).

Subsequently, I was involved in other GD-related studies delineating genotype–phenotype relationships, assessment of disease burden and mapping therapeutic profile in patients on enzyme therapy. Then as now, Robert J. Desnick, a leader in the field of lysosomal storage disorders (LSD), headed the Department of Human Genetics. In 1997, I moved to New York University to work with Edwin H. Kolodny whose interests included two other LSDs; specifically Tay-Sachs and Anderson-Fabry disease. The conjunction of these personalities and particular circumstances served as my introduction to the field, which to a large extent has defined my own professional life. These events were to also play a role in my personal life, as it enabled the happy occasion of meeting Derralynn A. Hughes, a hematologist at the Royal Free Hospital who was involved with caring for the London-based patients with GD and Anderson-Fabry disease. Derralynn and I were married in 2008, and at the time this book was written we have a daughter (Paloma).

Although my time at the Mayo Clinic was short, the individuals I met and the genuine spirit of mutual respect and high standard of patient care delivery I was to witness has formed a firm foundation, from which I was to draw the needed strength to confront the challenges I have subsequently had to deal with. In this regard, Virginia Michels was an excellent guide and teacher. More recently, Gilles Lyon, a French physician with whom Ed Kolodny and I co-authored a text entitled the *Neurology of Hereditary Metabolic and Molecular Diseases in Childhood* (2006), has been a source of inspiration.

I have been engaged in clinical practice and research in the field of LSDs for the past 20 years, and I was involved in several of the seminal trials to evaluate the safety and efficacy of various therapeutic options for several of these conditions. I believe this gives me a unique perspective, which I would now like to share with the readers of this book. Various investigators focus on different aspects in relation to LSDs, some are primarily clinicians and others do only basic scientific investigations. Thus, most books on the subject tend to be multi-authored, and can be variable in scope and depth. I have attempted to fill what I perceive as a gap in the existing literature: information in a single textbook which can serve as a concise guide not only for the novice, but for the expert as well whose focus or interest may be narrower than my personal experience.

Rapid progress is underway; thus, knowledge regarding pathophysiology and treatment of the LSDs is constantly undergoing revision. I have tried my best to present the most up-to-date information on the subject as I understand it. I would appreciate any effort by the reader to call attention to inaccuracies or outdated information, so this can be addressed in future editions of this monograph.

In closing, I would like to inscribe this book to my parents, Jovito C. Pastores and Annie H. McCarthy; both were equally devoted to my upbringing and education. My parents passed away within a span of one year, shortly before and after my wedding. What I am I know confidently has come from my parents; what I hope for and will become I pray my wife and daughter will enable.

Also, I would like to express my gratitude to the patients who have entrusted their care to me, and have given me the opportunity to develop my clinical skills. My interactions with the patients and their extended families have helped to enrich my life in several ways, because it has allowed me to learn of cultures and traditions that have not been part of my own upbringing. In entrusting their care to me, it is my fervent hope that I have met with their expectations.

Thus far, it has been a great adventure and I look forward to participating in future studies to elucidate the pathophysiology of LSDs and the development of treatment. Through the years I have interacted with and learned from several colleagues, and I am most grateful for the privilege and their mentorship.

Contents

List of Abbreviations

AAV	Adeno-associated virus
ABR	Auditory brain stem evoked response
ACE	Angiotensin-converting enzyme
AD	Alzheimer disease
AFD	Anderson-Fabry disease
AGAL	α-galactosidase A
AIMS	Alberta Infant Motor Scale
ALLO	Allopregnanolone
AMP	Adenosine monophosphate
AMPA	α-amino-3-hydroxyl-5-methyl-4-isoxazole-propionate
AMPK	AMP-activated protein kinase
ARSA	Arylsulfatase A
ATP	Adenosine triphosphate
BBB	Blood-brain-barrier
BDA	Bayh-Dole Act
BDNF	Brain-derived neurotrophic factor
BiP	Immunoglobulin binding protein/GRP78
BiPAP	Bi-level positive airway pressure
CADC	Cortical apparent diffusion coefficient
CCL18	Chemokine (C–C motif) ligand 18
CD3	Cluster of differentiation-3
Cho	Choline
CHO	Chinese hamster ovary
CHOP	C/EBP homology protein
CLN3	Ceroid-lipofuscinosis, neuronal-3

CNS	Central nervous system
CPAP	Continuous positive airway pressure
CRIM	Cross-reacting immunologic material
CSF	Cerebrospinal fluid
CTSD	Cathepsin D deficiency
CVS	Chorionic villus sampling
DGJ	Deoxygalactonojirimycin
DPP-IV	Dipeptidyl peptidase IV
EBP	Elastin binding protein
EMG	Electromyography
ER	Endoplasmic reticulum
ERG	Electroretinography
ERT	Enzyme replacement therapy
FAA	Functional activities assessment
FEV_1	Forced expiratory volume in the first second
FPSS	Functional performance scoring system
FVC	Forced vital capacity
GABA	Gamma-aminobutyric acid
GAG	Glycosaminoglycans
GALC	Galactocerebrosidase
GauSS-I	Gaucher disease Severity Score Index
Gb3	Globotriaosylceramide
GBA	Glucocerebrosidase
GD	Gaucher disease
GINA	Genetic Information Non-discrimination Act
GlcCer	Glucosylceramide
GluR2	Glutamate receptor subunit-2
HCII-TC	Heparin co-factor II-thrombin complex
HGSNAT	Heparan-α-glucosaminide N-acetyltransferase
HRQoL	Health-related quality of life
HS	Heparan sulphate
HSCT	Hematopoietic stem cell transplantation
I2S	Iduronate-2-sulfatase
IDUA	α-L-iduronidase
IL-1α	Interleukin-1α
ISSD	Infantile sialic acid storage disease

IT	Intrathecal
JNCL	Juvenile neuronal ceroid lipofuscinosis
JNK2	*c*-Jun *N*-terminal kinase-2
KS	Keratan sulfate
LCA	Leukocyte common antigen
LAMP2	Lysosomal-associated membrane protein-2
LIMP1	Lysosomal integral membrane protein-1
LINCL	Late-infantile neuronal ceroid lipofuscinosis
LOTS	Late-onset Tay-Sachs disease
LSD	Lysosomal storage disorder
LVH	Left ventricular hypertrophy
LVMi	Left ventricular mass index
lysoGb3	Deacylated globotriaosylceramide
MCOLN1	Mucolipin-1
M-CSF	Macrophage colony-stimulating factor
MEP	Maximal expiratory pressure
MIP	Maximal inspiratory pressure
ML-II/III/IV	Mucolipidosis type II/III/IV
MLC	Megalencephalic leukoencephalopathy with subcortical cysts
MLD	Metachromatic leukodystrophy
MOS	Medical outcomes study
MPS	Mucopolysaccharidosis
MRI	Magnetic resonance imaging
MRS	Magnetic resonance spectroscopy
MS	Mass spectroscopy
MSD	Multiple sulfatase deficiency
MSSI	Mainz Severity Score Index
mTOR	Mammalian target of rapamycin
MWT	Minute walk test
NAA	*N*-acetylaspartate
NCL	Neuronal ceroid lipofuscinosis
NCV	Nerve conduction velocity
NEU	Neuraminidase
NF-κB	Nuclear factor kappa-light-chain-enhancer of activated B cells

NFT	Neurofibrillary tangles
NPC	Niemann-Pick disease type C
NPD	Niemann-Pick disease
NIHF	Non-immune hydrops fetalis
ODA	Orphan Drug Act
OLP	Oligodendrocyte progenitor
PARC	Pulmonary and activation-regulated chemokine
PFT	Pulmonary function test
PPCA	Protective protein/cathepsin A
QMT	Quantitative muscle testing
REM	Rapid eye movement
ROS	Reactive oxygen species
SAP	Sphingolipid activator protein
Sap-B/C	Saposin B/C
SASD	Sialic acid storage disorders
SCMAS	Subunit C of mitochondrial ATP synthase
SD	Sandhoff disease
SDB	Sleep-disordered breathing
SELDI	Surface-enhanced laser desorption/ionization
SERCA	Sarco/Endoplasmic reticulum Ca^{2+}-ATPase
SPECT	Single photon emission computed tomography
SRT	Substrate reduction therapy
SSI	Severity score index
STAT	Signal transducers and activators of transcription
SUMF1	Sulfatase modifying factor 1
TIMP	Tissue inhibitor of metalloproteinase
TLC	Thin layer chromatography
TMS	Tandem mass spectrometry
TOF	Time-of-flight
TRAP	Tartrate-resistant acid phosphatase
TSD	Tay-Sachs disease
UCHL-1	Ubiquitin carboxyl-terminal esterase L1
UPR	Unfolded protein response
UPS	Ubiquitin-proteasome system
VEP	Visual evoked potential
VO_2	Maximal oxygen uptake

List of Figures

Vignette

The lysosomal storage disorder (LSD) widely known as *Gaucher disease* (*GD*) was first described in 1882 by a French dermatologist P.C.E. Gaucher. His patient was a 23-year-old woman with an enlarged spleen, attributed to an epithelioma. In 1965, R.O. Brady identified the underlying cause as an inborn error of metabolism, due to a deficiency of the lysosomal enzyme glucocerebrosidase. Almost 30 years later (1991), enzyme replacement therapy (ERT) was established as a safe and effective treatment for the condition. Therapy entailed the regular infusion of an enzyme preparation, initially derived from human placenta. Through the years, clinical investigations have enabled delineation of the clinical manifestations of *GD* (phenotype), recognition of neuronopathic and non-neuronopathic subtypes, and the mode of disease inheritance. Subsequently, several different causal mutations were identified, prompting examination of the relationship between genotype and phenotype. In 1994, a recombinant formulation of the enzyme, produced by transduction of Chinese hamster ovary cells, became available. Thus, a once potentially disabling condition is now one that can be effectively treated. Among remaining clinical challenges is the management of the neurologic problems in patients with the most severe subtypes of *GD*.

A Selection of Important Milestones

1907: F. Marchand reported the presence of a hyaline-like material in the so-called 'idiopathic splenomegaly of the *Gaucher type*' (type I non-neuronopathic form)

1924:   H. Lieb identified the storage material to be a cerebroside, which was characterized by H. Aghion to be glucocerebroside (rather than galactocerebroside, the material which accumulates in the brain tissue of patients with another LSD-*Krabbe disease*)

1927:   C. Oberling and P. Woringer recognized an infantile form of the disease, associated with acute neuronopathic involvement (type II *GD*)

1982:   G.A. Grabowski and colleagues reported prenatal diagnosis for *GD*, based on analysis of the enzyme activity in cultured amniocytes

1984:   E. Beutler and colleagues cloned and characterized both the functional glucocerebrosidase (*GBA*) gene and its closely linked pseudogene, which had been previously mapped to chromosome 1q21-q31 by A.J.J. Reuser and co-workers

1984:   E. Ginns reported the first case of bone marrow transplantation in an 8-year-old boy with type III *GD*

1988:   S. Karlsson and colleagues reported retroviral transfer of *GBA* into CD34[+] cells obtained from *GD* patients, and the *in vivo* detection of transduced cells.

Although significant progress has been made in the diagnosis and management of patients with *GD*, specific details regarding pathogenesis and the basis of phenotypic variability (which occurs even among patients with identical genotypes) are issues that remain to be more fully delineated. The introduction of alternative therapeutic options, such as substrate synthesis inhibition and the use of pharmacologic chaperones to enhance residual enzyme activity, offer the potential for an alternative, combinatorial or serial approach to patient care.

As evident from this brief description, the field of investigations for this lysosomal disorder, which in many ways serves as a paradigm for the others, has provided a bountiful harvest. But several questions remain. It is anticipated the discoveries made will provide new insights into more common clinical entities; for instance, search for the basis of increased risk for parkinsonism in patients and carriers of a glucocerebrosidase mutation may shed light on a common neurodegenerative disease encountered in the elderly.

Suggested Reading

Beutler E. Gaucher disease: Multiple lessons from a single gene disorder. *Acta Paediatr Suppl.* 2006;95(451):103–109.

Di Rocco M, Giona F, Carubbi F, Linari S, Minichilli F, Brady RO, Mariani G, Cappellini MD. A new severity score index for phenotypic classification and evaluation of responses to treatment in type I Gaucher disease. *Haematologica.* 2008;93(8):1211–1218.

Guggenbuhl P, Grosbois B, Chalès G. Gaucher disease. *Joint Bone Spine.* 2008; 75(2):116–124.

1

Introduction

The approach to the diagnosis and management of patients with lysosomal storage disorders (LSD) can be viewed as a model of specialized care delivery in the current era of medical practice. In particular, the introduction of disease-specific therapies, directed at the underlying biochemical defect and putative downstream mechanisms of disease, stands out as a practical application of advances made in translational research.

This introductory chapter describes aspects relating to the LSDs that have allowed its distinction from the broader group of inborn errors of metabolism. Topics discussed include major historical milestones that have brought us to where we find ourselves today, in terms of understanding causation and the clinical manifestations and natural history of individual clinical entities within this class of disease. Recent progress in the development of therapy, including currently available options and those under investigation, is also briefly presented.

The Lysosome and Storage Defects

Essentially the group of diseases classified as an LSD represents metabolic defects associated primarily with a disruption in the catabolism and/or transport of by-products of cellular turnover, coupled with the secondary consequences of the accumulation of incompletely metabolized substrates within particular cell types (Table 1.1). The principal organelle involved in the disease process is the lysosome, wherein the acidified environment (pH 5.0–5.5; actively maintained by a proton pump V type H^+ ATPase) and action of various hydrolases normally facilitate the

Table 1.1. The lysosomal storage disorders classified according to the relevant substrate involved.

Stored Substrate	Disease	Enzyme/Protein Deficiency	Gene Locus
A. Sphingolipids			
GM$_2$-gangliosides, glycolipids, globoside oligosaccharides	Tay-Sachs	α-subunit β-hexosaminidase	15q23-4
	GM$_2$-gangliosidosis (three types)*		
	Sandhoff disease	β-subunit β-hexosaminidase	5q13
	GM$_2$-gangliosidosis		
	GM$_2$-gangliosidosis, AB variant	G$_{M2}$ activator	5q32-33
GM$_1$-gangliosides, oligosaccharides, keratan sulfate, glycolipids	GM$_1$-gangliosidosis (three types)*	β-D-galactosidase	3p21.33
Sulphatides	Metachromatic leukodystrophy (MLD)	Arylsulphatase A (galactose-3-sulphatase)	22q13.31-qter
GM$_1$-gangliosides, sphingomyelin, glycolipids, sulphatide	MLD variant	Saposin B activator	10q21
Galactosylceramides	Krabbe disease	Galactocerebrosidase	14q31
α-galactosyl-sphingolipids, oligosaccharides	Anderson-Fabry disease	α-galactosidase A	Xq22
Glucosylceramide, globosides	Gaucher disease (GD) (three types)*	Glucocerebrosidase	1q21
Glucosylceramide, globosides	GD (variant)	Saposin C	10q21
Ceramide	Farber disease (seven types)	Acid ceramidase	8p22-21.2
Sphingomyelin	Niemann-Pick disease types A and B	Sphingomyelinase	11p15.1-15.4

(Continued)

Table 1.1. (*Continued*)

Stored Substrate	Disease	Enzyme/Protein Deficiency	Gene Locus
B. Mucopolysaccharidoses (Glycosaminoglycans)			
Dermatan sulphate (DS) and Heparan sulfate (HS)	MPS-I, Hurler, Scheie	*α*-L-iduronidase	4p16.3
	MPS-II, Hunter	Iduronate-2-sulphatase	Xq27.3-28
HS	MPS-IIIA, Sanfilippo A	Sulfamidase	17q25.3
	MPS-IIIB, Sanfilippo B	*α*-N-acetylglucosaminidase	17q21.1
	MPS-IIIC, Sanfilippo C	Acetyl CoA: *α*-glucosaminide-*N*-acetyltransferase	8p11
	MPS-IIID, Sanfilippo D	*N*-acetylglucosamine-6-sulfatase	12q14
Keratan sulphate (KS)	MPS-IVA, Morquio A	Galactosamine-6-sulphatase	16q24.3
	MPS-IVB, Morquio B	*β*-D-galactosidase	3p21.33
DS	MPS-VI, Maroteaux–Lamy	*N*-acetylgalactosamine-4-sulfatase	5q13-14
DS and HS	MPS-VII, Sly	*β*-D-glucuronidase	7q21.1-22
Hyaluronan	MPS-IX, Natowicz	Hyaluronidase	3p21.3
C. Glycogen			
Glycogen	Pompe, GSD II	*α*-D-glucosidase	17q25
Glycogen	Danon disease	Lysosomal associated membrane protein-2 (LAMP-2)	Xq24

Table 1.1. *(Continued)*

Stored Substrate	Disease	Enzyme/Protein Deficiency	Gene Locus
D. Oligosaccharides/ Glycopeptides			
α-mannoside	α-mannosidosis	α-mannosidase	19p13.2-q12
β-mannoside	β-mannosidosis	β-mannosidase	4q22-25
α-fucosides, glycolipids	α-fucosidosis	α-fucosidase	1p34.1-36.1
α-N-acetylgalactosaminide	Schindler/Kanzaki disease	α-N-acetylgalactosaminidase	22q13.1-13.2
Sialyloligosaccharides	Sialidosis	α-neuraminidase	6p21.3
Aspartylglucosamine	Aspartylglucosaminuria	Aspartylglucosaminidase	4q34-35
E. Multiple Enzyme Deficiencies			
Glycolipids, oligosaccharides	Mucolipidosis II (I-cell disease); mucolipidosis III (pseudo-Hurler polydystrophy) — three complementation groups	N-acetylglucosamine-1-phosphotransferase	4q21-q23; ML-III subtype C (a/b subunit 12q23.3; g subunit 16p)
Sulphatides, glycolipids, glycosaminoglycans	Galactosialidosis (protective protein/ cathepsin A)	Protective Protein/cathepsin A	20
	Multiple sulfatases (Austin disease)	SUMF-1	3p26

(Continued)

Table 1.1. *(Continued)*

Stored Substrate	Disease	Enzyme/Protein Deficiency	Gene Locus
F. Lipids			
Cholesterol esters	Wolman disease, CESD (cholesterol ester storage disease)	Acid lipase	10q23.2-q23.3
Cholesterol, sphingomyelin, GM_2-gangliosides	Niemann-Pick disease type C	NPC1; HE1	18q11-12; 14q24.3
G. Monosaccharides/Amino Acid Monomers			
Sialic acid, glucuronic acid	Salla, ISSD	Sialin	6q14-15
Cystine	Cystinosis	Cystinosin	17p13
H. Peptides			
Bone proteins	Pycnodysostosis	Cathepsin K	1q21
I. S-acylated Proteins			
Palmitoylated proteins	Infantile neuronal ceroid lipofuscinosis (NCL)	Palmitoyl-protein thioesterase	1p32
Pepstatin–insensitive lysosomal peptidase	Late-infantile NCL	Pepstatin–insensitive lysosomal peptides	11p15.5
Cathepsin D	Congenital NCL	Lysosomal cysteine protease	11p15.5

*Three types imply infantile, childhood and adulthood presentations.

processing of different macromolecules (substrates).[1] Lysosomal hydrolases frequently act in a sequential way, which may partly explain the
overlap in the nature of substrates stored and the associated clinical features (Figure 1.1).

Materials internalized by the cells rely on endocytosis and other
mechanisms (e.g., phagocytosis) to expedite entry into common endosomal structures (Figure 1.2). Ultimately the 'cargo' reaches the lysosome,

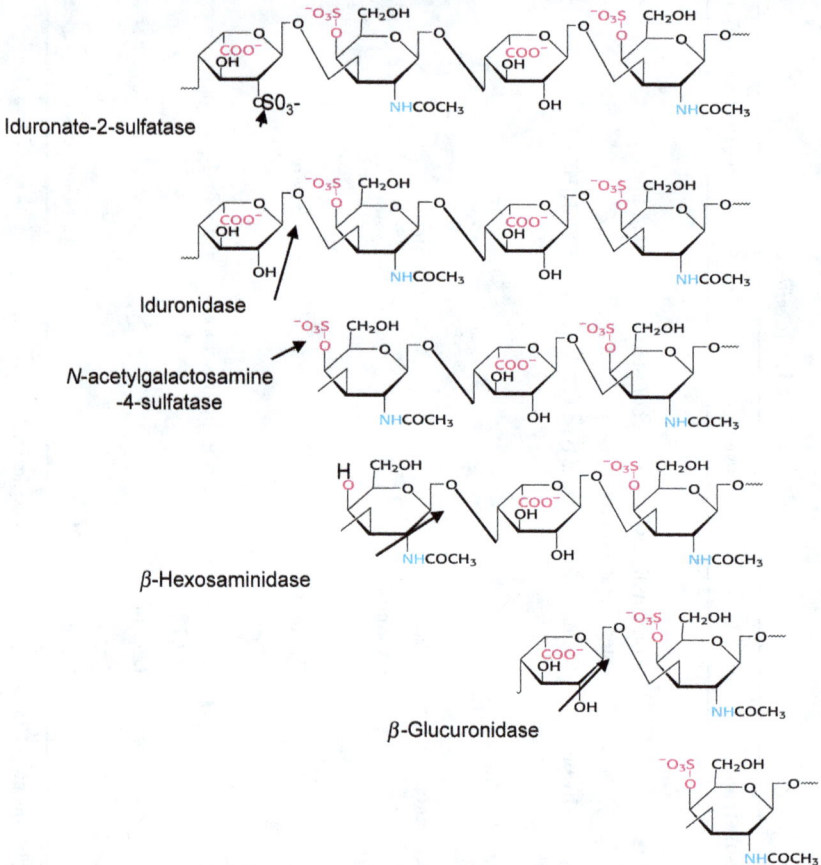

Figure 1.1. Schematic illustration of the sequential degradation of the glycosaminoglycan dermatan sulfate. Deficiency of distinct hydrolases gives rise to individual disorders,
the overlap in clinical presentations among the conditions in this group is partly explained
by the disruption of a common metabolic pathway.

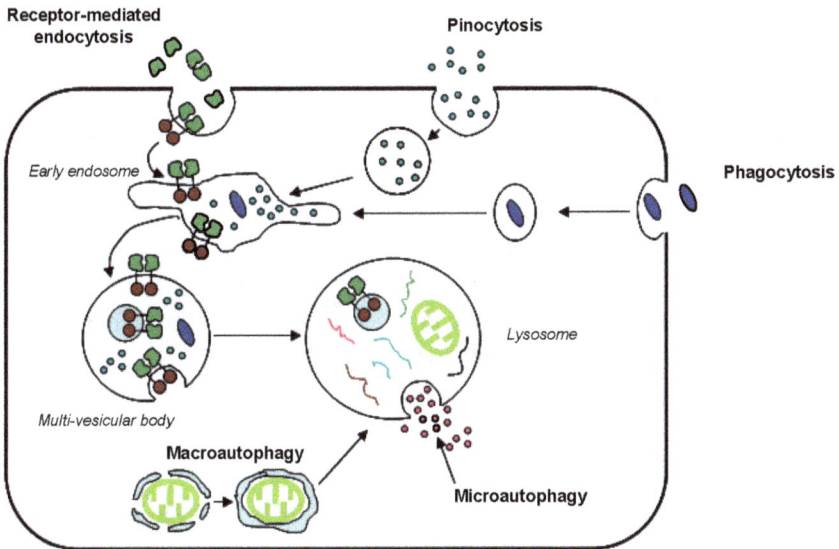

Figure 1.2. Schematic illustration of the endolysosomal system and the mechanisms involved in the delivery of exogenous and endogenous 'cargo' to the lysosome for processing.

which can be viewed as a central compartment in the cellular system for the breakdown and discharge or recycling of various substrates. The stability and integrity of the lysosomal limiting membrane is maintained with the assistance of highly glycosylated proteins, such as LAMP-1/2, that prevent lysosomal autodigestion.

Initial characterization of the lysosome was made by Christian DeDuve (circa 1955).[2] Coincidentally, it was another physician in the group at the *Universite Catholique de Louvain*, Henri-Géry Hers (c.1963), who described the enzyme (α-glucosidase) which is deficient in a glycogen storage disorder (*Pompe disease*), considered the first of the LSDs to be delineated as such. *Pompe disease* is named after the Dutch pathologist Johannes C. Pompe who in 1932 described a case of a 7-month-old infant with generalized muscle weakness and hypertrophic cardiomyopathy. Examination of the patient's cardiac tissue revealed glycogen deposits that were membrane-enclosed. This observation supported the concept of disease associated with lysosomal membrane enclosed-deposits, as distinct from conditions associated with organ infiltration by malignant cells or infectious agents. Eventually, it was recognized that the storage material represented incompletely degraded substrates that accumulated on account of an underlying enzyme deficiency or transport problem. These pivotal studies established the concept of lysosomal storage disorders, and provided a unifying framework for a diverse group of disorders discussed in greater detail in subsequent chapters.

Besides *Pompe disease* (*glycogen storage disorder type II*), several LSDs have been given an eponym in recognition of the physician/scientist who played a role in their seminal description (Table 1.2). *Salla disease* is unique in being named after a locale rather than an individual; this disorder was first described by P. Aula and colleagues in 1979, and named after a district in the Finnish Lapland. *Salla disease* is one of nearly 40 diseases (including two other LSDs, *aspartylglucosaminuria* and *infantile neuronal ceroid lipofuscinosis*) that make up the Finnish 'disease heritage'; a consequence of founder effect (i.e., shared identity by common descent).[3] A similar phenomenon is observed among the Ashkenazi Jews, in whom there is a high frequency of carriers for four LSDs, specifically, *Tay-Sachs disease, Gaucher disease, Niemann-Pick type A* and *mucolipidosis type IV*.[4]

To date, the LSDs encompass at least 50 different clinical entities. Initially, the individual disorders were grouped according to the chemical composition of the storage material, e.g., *sphingolipidoses, mucopolysaccharidoses, oligosaccharidoses*. More recently, these disorders have been clustered according to their underlying biochemical or molecular basis. In most, disease arises because of a deficiency of an enzyme or its co-factor, or because of a defect in a transport protein or other protein involved in the post-translational modification of the hydrolytic enzyme which precludes its functional maturation (a subject covered in more detail in Chapter 5).

Clinical Presentations and Diagnosis

By and large, the characteristic signs and symptoms of the individual LSDs reflect the cell types that are the principal sites of substrate deposits. Besides mechanical tissue disruption, investigations have revealed other pathogenic mechanisms, such as the activation of the endoplasmic reticulum

Table 1.2. Brief biographical sketches.

Designation	Year	Description Date	Biographical Notes
ANDERSON, William	1842–1900	1898	Born in London, UK; he was surgical registrar and demonstrator in anatomy at St. Thomas' Hospital, London
AUSTIN, James H.	1925–	1973	Born in the USA; studied Medicine at Harvard Medical School, Boston; trained in Neurology at the Neurological Institute, Columbia University, New York; Chair of the Department of Neurology, sequentially, at the University of Oregon Medical School and then at the University of Colorado Medical School
BATTEN, Frederick E.	1866–1918	1903	Born in Plymouth, England; studied Medicine at St. Bartholomew's Hospital, London; pathologist at the Hospital for Sick Children and physician at the National Hospital, Queens Square; regarded as father of British pediatric neurology
FABRY, Johannes	1860–1930	1898	Born in Germany; studied Medicine at St. Bartholomew's Hospital, London; dermatologist in Dortmund, Germany, trained at the Royal Clinic for Skin and Venereal disease in Bonn
FARBER, Sidney	1903–1973	1952	Born in Buffalo, New York, USA; studied Medicine at Harvard Medical School, Boston; was a pathologist at the Children's Hospital in Boston; became president of the American Association of Pathologists
GAUCHER, Phillipe C.E.	1854–1918	1882	Born in Champfleury, Nievre, France; dermatologist at the Hopital Saint-Antoine, Paris

(Continued)

Table 1.2. (*Continued*)

Designation	Year	Description Date	Biographical Notes
KRABBE, Knud	1885–1965	1913	Born in Denmark; Professor of Neurology and chief of service at the Community Hospital of Copenhagen; founded the *Acta Psychiatrica et Neurologica Scandinavia*
HUNTER, Charles	1873–1955	1917	Born in Auchterlass, Aberdeenshire, Scotland; studied Medicine at the University of Aberdeen; practiced as an internist in Winnipeg, Canada; taught at the Faculty of Medicine, University of Manitoba
HURLER, Gertrud (nee Zach)	1889–1965	1919	Born in Taberwiese, district of Rastenburg, Prussia; studied Medicine at the University of Munich; trained in Pediatrics at the Hauner Children's Hospital, and moved to private practice in Neuhausen
LAMY, Maurice	1895–1975	1963	Born in France; Professor of Pediatrics at the Hopital des Enfants Malades, Paris; co-organized the 4th International Congress of Human Genetics (ICHG) Paris
MAROTEAUX, Pierre	1926–	1963	Born in Versailles, France; studied Medicine at the University of Paris; director of the National Center of Scientific Research, Hopital des Enfants Malades, Paris; co-organized 4th ICHG
MORQUIO, Luis	1867–1935	1929	Born in Montevideo, Uruguay; studied Medicine at the University of Munich; Professor of Pediatrics at the University of Montevideo
NIEMANN, Albert	1880–1921	1920	Born in Berlin, Germany; Professor of Pediatrics at the University Children's Clinic, and Director of The Infant's Home at Berlin-Halensee
PICK, Ludwig	1868–1944	1914	Born in Landsberg, Germany; Professor of Pathology at the University of Berlin; died in the concentration camp at Theresienstadt

(*Continued*)

Table 1.2. *(Continued)*

Designation	Year	Description Date	Biographical Notes
POMPE, Johannes C.	1901–1945	1932	Born in Holland; Pathologist; executed by the Nazi's for his role in the resistance
SACHS, Bernard	1858–1944	1887	Born in Baltimore, Maryland (USA); Professor of Neurology at the Polyclinic, Mount Sinai & Bellevue, New York
SANDHOFF, Konrad	1939–	1965	Born in Berlin, Germany; degree in chemistry at the Ludwig Maximillian University; headed the Department of Neurochemistry, Max Planck Institute for Psychiatry, Munich; Professor of Biochemistry, University of Bonn
SCHEIE, Harold	1909–1990	1962	Born in North Dakota (USA); trained in Ophthalmology and was Professor at the Department of Ophthalmology in University of Pennsylvania
SLY, William	1932–	1973	Born in the USA; studied Medicine at St. Louis University, and trained at the NIH and CNRS Laboratory in France; Professor and Chair, Departments of Biochemistry and Molecular Biology, St. Louis University School of Medicine
TAY, Warren	1843–1927	1881	Born in Plymouth, England; studied Medicine at London Hospital; practiced as an ophthalmologist, pediatrician, and surgeon
WOLMAN, Moshe	1914–	1984	Born in Warsaw, Poland; Professor and Chairman of Pathology at the University of Tel-Aviv, Israel

stress response, inflammatory and/or apoptotic cascade. At this time, details of disease mechanisms that promote tissue damage and organ dysfunction are incompletely understood.

Several clinical manifestations, such as hepatosplenomegaly, coarse facial features and skeletal dysplasia, can serve as an important clue which should lead to consideration of the patient's problems as likely to be due to an LSD (see Chapter 2). Of note, on presentation, especially in a young child, the diagnosis can be missed, especially when the family history is uninformative. Broad heterogeneity in clinical presentation and the wide variability in age at onset and rate of disease progression are additional factors that can lead to significant delay in diagnosis. Diagnostic confirmation necessitates biochemical and/or molecular genetic testing (Chapter 3).

The molecular basis of a majority of the LSDs has been identified. Characterization of the gene defects in affected individual has revealed the occurrence of several distinct mutations. Although this phenomenon partly explains differences in disease severity, extensive studies to examine the relationship between genotype (gene defect) and phenotype (clinical expression) have often shown the lack of perfect concordance. However, in general, deleterious (null) mutations that give rise to a complete or severe enzyme deficiency tend to be associated with an earlier age of disease onset and a graver clinical course. Missense mutations associated with residual enzyme activity usually lead to attenuated clinical subtypes. Investigations of the factors that may influence disease expression are subjects of great interest and are further explored in Chapter 5.

In another group of inborn metabolic errors, the peroxisomal disorders, testing of plasma/serum levels of a single analyte (i.e., very long-chain fatty acids, VLCFA) can point to the diagnosis. Unfortunately, such is not the case with LSDs, in which the diagnosis when suspected often necessitates testing for the presence of excess substrates in body fluids or the activity of several different enzymes in blood or tissues. Thus, it is helpful to have some familiarity with the principal signs and symptoms of particular entities or subgroup of LSDs, so that appropriate testing can be undertaken. Population and newborn screening strategies for LSDs are currently under consideration. This topic and a discussion of methods used to confirm the diagnosis are reviewed in Chapter 3.

Disease Burden and Therapeutic Considerations

The LSDs are defined by regulatory agencies as 'orphan' disorders, that is, affecting individuals numbering < 200,000 in the United States (US), or no more than 5/10,000 in Europe. In the United States, therapeutic options for the LSDs have and are being developed, pursuant to two landmark legislation: the Bayh-Dole Act (BDA, 1980) and the Orphan Drug Act (ODA, 1983). Essentially, these acts of congress enabled universities to patent their discoveries and license them to private corporations (BDA); in turn, the biotech companies have received several incentives (including the potential of fast-track approval and marketing exclusivity) to stimulate the development of medical drugs and devices for rare disorders (ODA).[5] Patient advocacy groups have played a major part in upholding the enactment of these and related legislation, including the more recent Genetic Information Non-discrimination Act (GINA) of 2007–2008.

With the introduction of therapy for LSDs (reviewed in Chapter 6), mainly consisting of the infusion of the relevant recombinant formulation of the deficient enzyme, several guidelines for measuring disease burden or stage and monitoring therapeutic outcomes have been developed (Chapter 4). In practice, the choice of clinical investigations to assess disease severity is usually driven by knowledge of the major organs that can be involved in particular conditions. With advances in disease management and the resultant increase in patient survival, there is a need to ensure continuity of care by physicians, especially when dealing with major life transitions. This can be a challenge, particularly for those trained in 'adult medicine' who may not fully appreciate the medical and psychological needs of affected individuals with an LSD, as historically these patients were managed primarily by pediatricians and metabolic specialists.[6] The complex nature of the disease processes encountered in patients with an LSD necessitates care by a multidisciplinary team, ideally at designated 'centers of excellence'.

As the number of study patients in the various clinical trials was small, the issue of optimal dose and frequency of exogenous enzyme administration and other management considerations remain open subjects for debate.[7,8] Meanwhile, other therapeutic options, including the use of small molecules that either inhibit substrate synthesis or serve as a pharmacologic chaperone, have been developed or are under investigation.

Moreover, there are on-going pre-clinical investigations involving gene therapy and stem cell transplantation for the LSDs (covered in Chapter 6). These developments are anticipated to lead to significant improvement in patient survival and quality of life, for diseases that until recently could only be dealt by palliative measures.

Screening and Genetic Counseling Issues

Although individual disorders are rare, the LSDs collectively account for a significant proportion of the population that is chronically ill as a consequence of a genetic disease (Table 1.3). Unfortunately, the diagnosis and

Table 1.3.   Disease incidence for selected LSDs.*

Disease	Incidence
• Aspartylglycosaminuria	1 in 3643 (Finland)
• Cystinosis	1 in 281,000
• Anderson-Fabry disease	1 in 117,000
• Gaucher disease	1 in 59,000 (non-Jewish population)
• Krabbe disease	1 in 201,000[†]
• Metachromatic leukodystrophy	1 in 121,000[‡]
• Mucopolysaccharidosis (MPS)	Collectively 1 in 25,000
• MPS-I Hurler syndrome	1 in 111,000
• MPS-II Hunter syndrome	1 in 136,000
• MPS-III Sanfilippo syndrome	Collectively 1 in 63,700[§]
• MPS-VI Maroteaux-Lamy syndrome	1 in 300,000
• Multiple sulfatase deficiency	1 in 1.4 million
• Neuronal ceroid lipofuscinosis	Collectively 1 in 12,500
• Niemann-Pick A/B	1 in 249,000
• Niemann-Pick C	1 in 230,000
• Pompe disease	1 in 201,000

*Mainly drawn from Meikle PJ, Hopwood JJ, Claque AE, Carey WF. *JAMA* 1999 January 20;281(3): 249–254.

[†]1 in 25,000 for *early infantile form* in Sweden.

[‡]1/2,520 live births in Navajo Indians of the Southwestern United States, 1/75 live births in a small Jewish community in Habban, Yemen.

[§]MPS IIIA is the most common subtype in Northern Europe, whereas MPS IIIB is more prevalent in Southern Europe.

management of afflicted patients remains a major challenge, particularly for those with clinical variants associated with central nervous system involvement. Several advances, including methods for carrier detection and prenatal and pre-implantation genetic diagnosis, are providing individuals at risk with options in the course of family planning. However, in most cases the inability to accurately predict long-term prognosis is a confounding factor in the counseling of families.

Rapid scientific progress has enabled the development of an increasing number of therapeutic options. Symptomatic and directed therapies have resulted in increased survival, with significant improvement in quality of life in a significant proportion of treated patients. Keys to good outcome include early diagnosis and timely intervention. Meanwhile, intensive investigation of disease mechanisms is anticipated to provide additional targets for pharmacologic intervention to enable optimal health outcomes.

References

1. Reuser AJ, Drost MR. Lysosomal dysfunction, cellular pathology and clinical symptoms: Basic principles. *Acta Paediatr Suppl.* 2006;95(451):77–82.

2. de Duve C. The lysosome turns fifty. *Nat Cell Biol.* 2005;7(9):847–849.

3. Peltonen L, Jalanko A, Varilo T. Molecular genetics of the Finnish disease heritage. *Hum Mol Genet.* 1999;8(10):1913–1923.

4. Ostrer H. A genetic profile of contemporary Jewish populations. *Nat Rev Genet.* 2001;2(11):891–898.

5. Graul AI. Promoting, improving and accelerating the drug development and approval processes. *Drug News Perspect.* 2009;22(1):30–38.

6. Schwarz M, Wendel U. Inborn errors of metabolism (IEM) in adults. A new challenge to internal medicine. *Med Klin (Munich).* 2005;100(9):547–552.

7. Pastores GM, Barnett NL. Current and emerging therapies for the lysosomal storage disorders. *Expert Opin Emerg Drugs.* 2005;10(4):891–902.

8. Sidransky E, Pastores GM, Mori M. Dosing enzyme replacement therapy for Gaucher disease: Older, but are we wiser? *Genet Med.* 2009;11(2):90–91.

Vignette

In 1919, while training in Pediatrics, Gertrude Hurler described two patients with corneal clouding, short stature (associated with skeletal dysplasia) and mental retardation. The patients' clinical features were noted to be similar to two brothers whose medical histories were presented by Charles Hunter at a meeting of the Royal Society of Medicine in London in 1917. Subsequently, these patients were found to have excessive mucopolysaccharides (glycosaminoglycans) in their urine; an observation that led to their categorization as having a biochemical disorder, designated *mucopolysaccharidosis* (*MPS*).

The concept of disease as resulting from an inborn error of metabolism was developed by Archibald Garrod, and first introduced in a 1908 Croonian Lecture and at the Huxley Lecture given at Charing Cross Hospital in London in 1927. The notion encompasses defects of amino and organic acid metabolism, peroxisomal disorders and lysosomal storage disorders (LSD). In this scheme, the *MPS* disorders represent a subgroup of the LSDs.

With identification of distinct enzyme deficiencies as the basis for the *MPS* disorder, numerical designations were given to each entity based on the chronologic order of their description. *Hurler syndrome*, the prototypical *MPS* which is caused by a deficiency of α-L-iduronidase, became known as *MPS-I*, and *Hunter syndrome* (iduronate-2-sulfatase deficiency) was designated *MPS-II*. Several mutations have been identified in the relevant genes, responsible for *MPS-I* or *II*, which segregate as an autosomal recessive and X-linked trait, respectively.

Suggested Reading

Clarke LA. The mucopolysaccharidoses: a success of molecular medicine. *Expert Rev Mol Med*. 2008 (January 18);10:e1.

Hunter C. A rare disease in two brothers. *Proc R Soc Med*. 1917;10:104–116.

Hurler G. A type of multiple degeneration that mainly affects the skeletal system. *Z Kinderheilkd*. 1919;24(5–6):220–234.

2

Clinical Perspectives

The diagnosis of a lysosomal storage disorder (LSD) is often suspected based on clinical features, age at onset and disease course, as well as family history, when informative. The LSDs defer clinically from other inborn errors of metabolism, such as the organic acidemias or defects of mitochondrial function leading to energy depletion; disorders that are usually associated with 'intoxication-type' symptoms. In these latter metabolic disorders, there can be acute decompensation with encephalopathy and altered mental status, problems that can be related to the intake of certain foods or a period of prolonged fasting. In contrast, the LSDs are often insidious processes and although there are acute disease subtypes, clinical manifestations often develop over weeks and months rather than hours or days.

The diagnosis of an LSD is often missed on presentation, particularly in those with a negative family history. Diagnosis can also be delayed, especially during the initial stages, when signs and symptoms may be limited and non-specific.[1] These scenarios are not uncommon, especially in subtypes associated with primary central nervous system (CNS) involvement, when there are no visceral or skeletal signs that serve as a clue to the presence of a storage defect. Affected individuals usually present to the pediatrician or geneticist for evaluation of developmental delay or mental retardation, triggering an initial work up that may include clinical investigations, such as complete blood count, liver and kidney function tests, urinalysis, amino and organic acid profiling, and chromosome analysis (karyotyping). Although helpful in excluding certain disorders, these tests do not yield hints to an LSD diagnosis, which is critical for establishing a treatment plan, including the counseling of relatives about their potential of being a carrier of the gene defect and its reproductive implications.

The biochemical nature of the storage material and primary sites of tissue deposition define the clinical features associated with individual disorders. Thus, LSDs associated with the storage of gangliosides and sulfatides, which are major components of neuronal membranes, lead primarily to neuropathology. Similarly, storage of keratan sulfate (KS), a major constituent of cartilage and the cornea, partly explain the skeletal dysplasia and corneal opacities associated with the *mucopolysacchari-doses* *(MPS)*. Familiarity with the clinical signs and symptoms of the different clinical variants is critical to enabling accurate diagnosis, which can be confirmed by appropriate biochemical and/or molecular assays (described in Chapter 3).

Extra-neurologic systemic manifestations that should lead to consideration of LSD include coarse facial features, cardiomyopathy, hepatosplenomegaly, skeletal dysplasia or renal insufficiency. At onset, it may not be apparent that multiple systems are involved. Thus, a high index of suspicion must be maintained, particularly when clinical problems develop and are persistent or progressive, and remain unexplained. Tables 2.1 and 2.2 list common signs and symptoms encountered in the various LSDs.

Knowledge of the typical age at onset for the most common variants of the LSDs is an important factor in generating a list of potential diagnoses for a patient with a suspected storage disorder (Table 2.3). However, it is essential to note that most individual disorders are associated with a wide range in ages at presentation, from birth to the fifth decade, or later. Thus, while most clinical subtypes are evident during early to late childhood, one should not dismiss consideration of an LSD as the basis of clinical problems that develop later on in life. Indeed, diagnosis is often missed in those with an adult-onset LSD, in whom gait problems, cognitive impairment and psychiatric or behavioral changes may be the dominant complaint.

Manifesting Signs and Corresponding Diagnostic Entities

Conceptually, the various clinical presentations of individual disorders can be viewed as falling within a spectrum, partly attributable to differences

Table 2.1. Extra-neurologic clinical manifestations reported in patients with an LSD.

Non-immune hydrops fetalis	*Cytopenia (anemia, thrombocytopenia)*	*Hepatosplenomegaly*
• Disseminated lipogranulomatosis (Farber disease)	• Gaucher disease	• Gaucher disease
	• Niemann-Pick disease	• Mucopolysaccharidoses
• Galactosialidosis (neuraminidase deficiency)	• Wolman disease (acanthocytosis)	• Niemann-Pick disease A and B
• Gaucher disease		• Niemann-Pick C (cholestatic jaundice)
• G$_{M1}$-gangliosidosis	*Interstitial lung disease*	• Oligosaccharidoses
• Infantile free sialic acid storage disease (ISSD)	• Gaucher disease	• Wolman disease and cholesterylester storage disease
	• Niemann-Pick disease	
• Mucolipidosis II (I-cell disease)	*Obstructive airway disease*	*Nephrolithiasis*
• Mucopolysaccharidosis types IV and VII	• Anderson-Fabry disease	• Cystinuria
	• Mucopolysacc haridoses	
• Niemann-Pick disease type C	*Cardiomyopathy*	*Proteinuria*
• Sialidosis type I	• Anderson-Fabry disease (arrhythmia, conduction abnormalities)	• Anderson-Fabry disease
• Wolman disease	• MPS (valvular disease)	• SASD (nephrotic syndrome)
	• Pompe disease (hypotonia)	

in the causal mutations (i.e., allelic heterogeneity). Deleterious gene defects that result in a complete or drastic reduction in protein function usually lead to severe subtypes, often associated with an early- or late-infantile onset and neurodegenerative features. On the other hand, disease caused by mutations associated with residual enzyme/protein activity tend to manifest at a later age and follow a relatively attenuated course.

Generalized: Non-immune hydrops fetalis

Neonatal presentation is infrequent, although several LSDs may manifest in the first few weeks of life with non-immune hydrops fetalis (NIHF) or 'collodion skin' (Table 2.4). In a study of 75 cases of NIHF, the diagnosis of definite and probable LSD was made in four and two instances, respectively, an incidence of 5.3 to 8%.[2] As these cases are usually associated with a high mortality rate, it is essential to proceed with the

Table 2.2. Neurologic clinical manifestations reported in patients with an LSD.

Cherry-red spot, Optic atrophy, Visual loss
- Galactosialidosis
- G_{M1}-gangliosidosis
- Infantile free sialic acid storage disease (ISSD)
- Mucolipidosis II (I-cell disease)
- Mucopolysaccharidosis types IV (MPS IV) and VII (MPS VII)
- Neuronal ceroid lipofuscinosis
- Niemann-Pick disease type A
- Sialidosis type I
- Sandhoff disease
- Tay-Sachs disease

Retinitis pigmentosa
- Neuronal ceroid lipofuscinosis
- Danon disease

Corneal opacities (clouding)
- I-cell disease (ML-II)
- Mucolipidosis IV (ML-IV)
- MPS-I, IV, VI
- Oligosaccharidosis (late-onset α-mannosidosis)
- Anderson-Fabry disease

Lenticular opacities (cataracts)
- Oligosaccharidosis (sialidosis, α-mannosidosis)
- Anderson-Fabry disease

Ophthalmoplegia (Abnormal eye movements), Nystagmus
- Gaucher disease III
- Niemann-Pick C
- Salla disease

Leukodystrophy
- Krabbe disease
- MLD
- Anderson-Fabry disease*
- Salla disease

Myoclonic seizures
- Galactosialidosis
- Gaucher disease III
- G_{M2}-gangliosidosis
- Neuronal ceroid lipofuscinosis
- Niemann-Pick C

- Oligosaccharidosis (α-N-acetylgalactosaminidase deficiency, fucosidosis, Sialidosis type I)

Deafness[†]
- Anderson-Fabry disease
- Galactosialidosis
- Gaucher disease type II
- I-cell disease
- MPS-I, II, IV
- Oligosaccharidosis (α- and β-mannosidosis)
- Metachromatic leukodystrophy
- Infantile Pompe disease

(Continued)

Table 2.2.   (*Continued*)

Macrocephaly	• Neuronal ceroid lipofuscinosis	• ML IV
• Tay-Sachs disease		• MLD
• Sandhoff disease		• Neuronal ceroid lipofuscinosis
• Krabbe disease	*Cerebrovascular or stroke-like episodes and other vascular events (e.g., Raynaud's phenomenon)*	• Niemann-Pick C
Peripheral neuropathy		• Salla disease
• Krabbe disease	• Anderson-Fabry disease	• Sialidosis I
• MLD (spastic paraplegia)		
• Multiple sulfatase deficiency	*Ataxia*	*Extrapyramidal signs*
	• Galactosialidosis	• Gaucher disease III
Cortical atrophy	• Gaucher disease III	• G$_{M1}$-gangliosidosis (adult form)
• Late stage of G$_{M1}$- and G$_{M2}$-gangliosidosis (cerebellar atrophy)	• G$_{M1}$-gangliosidosis	• Late-onset G$_{M2}$-gangliosidosis
	• Late-onset G$_{M2}$-gangliosidosis (cerebellar hypoplasia)	• Krabbe disease
• MLD		• Niemann-Pick C
• I-cell disease	• Krabbe disease	• Oligosaccharidosis

Dementia, Psychosis
• Anderson-Fabry disease
• Gaucher disease III
• G$_{M1}$-gangliosidosis
• Late-onset G$_{M2}$-gangliosidosis
• Krabbe disease
• MLD
• MPS-III (Sanfilippo disease)
• Neuronal ceroid lipofuscinosis
• Niemann-Pick C

*Signal abnormalities consistent with leukoaraiosis.

†Conductive, sensorineural, or a combination, with involvement of cochlea and CNS dysfunction.

Table 2.3. Presenting clinical manifestations associated with selected LSDs, delineated based on age of onset.

Age at Onset	Presenting Signs and Associated Clinical Features
First Year	
Farber disease (ceramidase deficiency)	Hoarseness, vomiting, swollen joints, subcutaneous nodules, lymphadenopathy, foamy macrophages
Fucosidosis, type I	Slow development, with rapid progression leading to decerebrate rigidity, coarse facies, vacuolated lymphocytes
Gaucher disease, type II	Failure to thrive, hepatosplenomegaly, brain stem signs, spasticity
G_{M1}-gangliosidosis, type I	Slow development, increased startle, hepatosplenomegaly, gibbus deformity
G_{M2}-gangliosidosis, Sandhoff variant	Slow development, increased startle, cherry-red spot, splenomegaly
Hunter disease	Coarse facies, stiff joints, heart murmur
Hurler disease	Coarse facies, stiff joints
α-mannosidosis	Slow development, coarse facies, hepatosplenomegaly, moderate to severe MR
Mucolipidosis II	Wizened face at birth, gingival hyperplasia, stiff joints
Mucolipidosis IV	Slow development, corneal clouding
Mucosulfatidosis	Slow development, coarse facies
Neuronal ceroid lipofuscinosis, infantile type	Slow development, poor vision, seizures
Niemann-Pick disease, A	Slow development, hepatosplenomegaly, cherry-red spot
Sanfilippo disease	Coarse facies (subtle), stiff joints, severe mental retardation
Sialic acid storage disease	Slow development, hepatosplenomegaly, coarse facies
Sialidosis type II, late-infantile	Slow development, coarse facies, hepatomegaly
Tay-Sachs disease	Loss of interest in environment, exaggerated startle response, rapid deterioration
Wolman disease	Vomiting, diarrhea, hepatosplenomegaly, calcified adrenals

(*Continued*)

Table 2.3. (*Continued*)

Age at Onset	Presenting Signs and Associated Clinical Features
Second Year	
Aspartylglucosaminuria	Slow development, delayed or absent speech, coarse facies, aggressive behavior
Fucosidosis, type II	Slow neurologic deterioration, speech problems, angiokeratoma
G_{M1}-gangliosidosis, type II	Slow development, increased startle
Maroteaux-Lamy syndrome	Coarse facies, stiff joints, corneal clouding
Morquio syndrome	Dwarfism, skeletal abnormalities, loose joints in the wrist
Mucolipidosis III	Stiff hands and shoulders
Neuronal ceroid lipofuscinosis, late infantile type	Seizures, myoclonus, decreased vision, intellectual deterioration
Niemann-Pick disease, B	Hepatosplenomegaly, interstitial lung disease
Sialidosis type II	Walking difficulties, seizures, myoclonus, mental deterioration, macular cherry-red spot
Childhood	
Cholesteryl ester storage disease	Hepatomegaly, increased plasma cholesterol and triglycerides
Galactosialidosis	Delayed motor development, mental retardation, seizures, myoclonus, coarse facial features
Gaucher disease, type I	Splenomegaly, anemia, thrombocytopenia, osteopenia, osteonecrosis
Maroteaux-Lamy syndrome, mild	Short stature, limitation in joint range of motion, coarse facies, corneal clouding, lumbar lordosis, normal intelligence, cardiac valvular disease
Neuronal ceroid lipofuscinosis, juvenile type	Blindness, seizures, intellectual deterioration
Niemann-Pick disease, chronic neuropathic form (types B and C)	Tetraparesis, intellectual deterioration, hepatomegaly, ataxia
Scheie disease	Claw hands, short stature

(*Continued*)

Table 2.3. (*Continued*)

Age at Onset	Presenting Signs and Associated Clinical Features
Adolescence	
Cherry-red spot myoclonus syndrome, sialidosis type I	Unexpected falls, seizures, cherry-red macula, corneal clouding
Gaucher disease, type III	Splenomegaly, seizures, myoclonus, osteopenia, osteonecrosis
G_{M2}-gangliosidosis, late-onset	Dysarthria, walking difficulties due to spastic paraparesis, cerebellar ataxia
Adulthood	
Gaucher disease, type I	Splenomegaly, thrombocytopenia, osteonecrosis
Anderson-Fabry disease	Proteinuria, renal insufficiency, cardiomyopathy, stroke
G_{M2}-gangliosidosis, late onset	Gait problems, proximal muscle weakness, ataxia, psychosis, manic-depressive illness
Maroteaux-Lamy syndrome, mild	Short stature, coarse facies, corneal clouding, compressive myelopathy
NCL, Kufs disease	Dementia, behavioral disturbances, epilepsy, ataxia
Pompe disease, adult type (acid maltase myopathy)	Proximal muscle weakness (limb-girdle myopathy), with intercostal and diaphragm involvement (leading to respiratory insufficiency)

collection of appropriate samples for analysis (see Chapter 3), after other more common entities such as congenital heart problems and genetic dermatoses have been excluded. Diagnosis of an LSD enables counseling on the uniformly severe course of the disease in this context, which may help assuage parental frustration, often derived from the perception that 'not enough is being done for my child'. In this situation, the family may be guided as to the need for certain diagnostic procedures and interventions that may not only be invasive but also would not have a significant influence on outcome. This way, efforts can be focused

Table 2.4. Disorders associated with non-immune hydrops fetalis and additional features.

• Disseminated lipogranulomatosis (Farber disease)	Painful joint swelling and deformities; dysphonia (hoarse cry); dyspnea; onset usually before age of 4 months
• Galactosialidosis (neuraminidase deficiency)	Cerebellar ataxia; myoclonus; visual failure; onset by late childhood or adolescence
• Gaucher disease	Anemia, thrombocytopenia, hepatosplenomegaly, neuronopathic forms: opisthotonus, seizures
• G_{M1}-gangliosidosis	Coarse facial features, corneal clouding, hepatomegaly, skeletal dysplasia, learning disability, myoclonus
• Infantile free sialic acid storage disease (ISSD)	Coarse facies, fair complexion, hepatosplenomegaly, and severe psychomotor retardation, nephrotic syndrome
• Mucolipidosis II (I-cell disease)	Coarse facies, short stature, kyphoscoliosis, umbilical and inguinal hernias
• Mucopolysaccharidosis types IV and VII	Short stature, skeletal dysplasia
• Niemann-Pick disease type C	Ataxia, swallowing problems, supranuclear gaze palsy, splenomegaly
• Sialidosis type II	Hepatomegaly and skeletal dysplasia, macular cherry-red spot, punctate lenticular opacities
• Wolman disease	Vomiting, diarrhea, hepatosplenomegaly, calcified adrenals

towards delivery of comfort and sustenance to the child. At the appropriate time, families will require counseling regarding future pregnancies, and options that are available to deal with the risk of recurrence.

Head, eyes, nose, ears and throat involvement

In the first few months of life, dysmorphic facial features reminiscent of those encountered in the *MPS* may be noted in patients with *I-cell disease* and the *infantile form of G_{M1}-gangliosidosis*. In *MPS* disorders, the distinctive facial features (frontal bossing, coarse hair and thickened skin and eyebrows) become evident later in infancy (usually between 6 and 18 months of life) or later in childhood (Figure 2.1). Characteristic

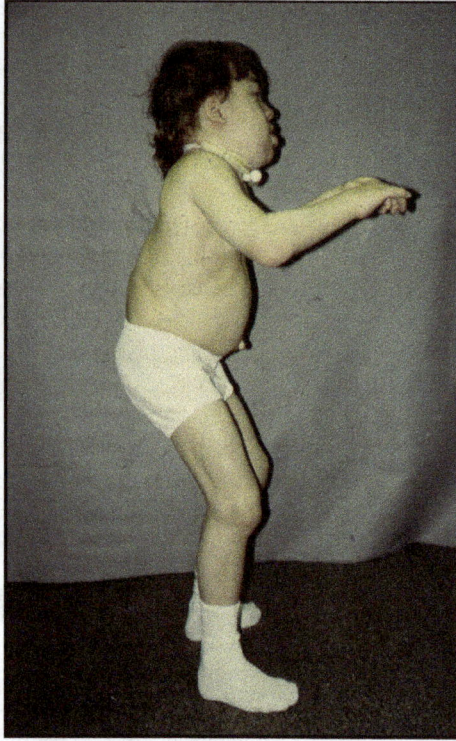

Figure 2.1.   Characteristic features of *MPS-I* in a child: thickened coarse hair, thick lips, short neck, gibbus deformity, joint contractures, and umbilical hernia.

findings in affected cases may also include a large and prominent tongue, broad and thickened gingiva and wide-spaced peg-shaped teeth. These features and other manifestations encountered in the *MPS* may also be seen in the *glycoproteinoses* (*oligosaccharidoses*), although they tend to be subtle.

Macrocephaly as a consequence of megalencephaly, in the absence of dysmorphic facial features and organomegaly, is encountered in infancy in patients with G_{M2}-*gangliosidosis* (*Tay-Sachs* and *Sandhoff disease*) and *globoid cell leukodystrophy* (*Krabbe disease*). In these patients, there is often rapid disease progression, with spasticity, feeding problems and premature death. In later onset forms of these disorders, patients display other neurologic problems such as ataxia; additionally, psychiatric problems may be an initial presentation in these cases.

Children with *aspartylglycosaminuria* tend to be tall and have macro-cephaly, but middle aged patients are microcephalic and have short stature.[3]

Macrocephaly is also noted in later infancy or early childhood in patients with *MPS*, associated with developmental delay and behavioral problems. Coarse facial features, organomegaly and skeletal dysplasia are other features of this diagnosis.

Communicating hydrocephalus is encountered in the *MPS*, as a con-sequence of impairment in CSF absorption with accumulation of glycosaminoglycans (GAGs) in the pia-arachnoid.[4] Spinal cord compres-sion may also develop in *MPS* patients, secondary to pachymeningitis; following the build-up of GAGs in the dura mater, usually involving the cervical spine region. In these patients, cord compression is often signaled by development of weakness in the lower extremities, with brisk reflexes and gait problems.

Corneal clouding, which can lead to impairment in visual acuity, is a prominent *MPS* features, except for type II disease (*Hunter syndrome*). In *Anderson-Fabry disease (AFD)* and *fucosidosis*, lenticular opacities can be detected by slit lamp examination. There is turtuosity of conjunctival blood vessels; however, *AFD* patients do not have overt visual problems, except in those who experience a stroke, which can manifest with vertigo and hemiplegia.[5] Corneal dystrophy has also been described in *mucolipi-dosis type IV (ML-IV)*, an LSD associated with developmental delay.

Visual loss secondary to retinal degeneration may develop in children with *MPS, ML-IV*, neuronal ceroid lipofuscinosis (*NCL*) and *oligosaccha-ridoses* (e.g., *sialidosis*). Patients with *Danon disease*, caused by mutations in *LAMP2*, have been described to have peripheral pigmentary retinopathy, lens changes, myopia, an abnormal electroretinogram and visual field defects.[6] Progressive visual loss, associated with polymyoclonus and seizures, develop in late childhood or adolescence in patients with *sialido-sis*.[7] The cherry-red spot can be found in *Tay-Sachs, Niemann-Pick A, sialidosis* and *Farber's lipogranulomatosis* (Figure 2.2; Table 2.5).[7,8] Associated clinical problems enable distinction of specific LSD subtype.

Hearing problems, caused by stiffness and deformity of the auricular bones of the middle ear resulting in conductive hearing loss, occur in the *MPS* and *oligosaccharidoses*. Unilateral or bilateral hearing loss is also a

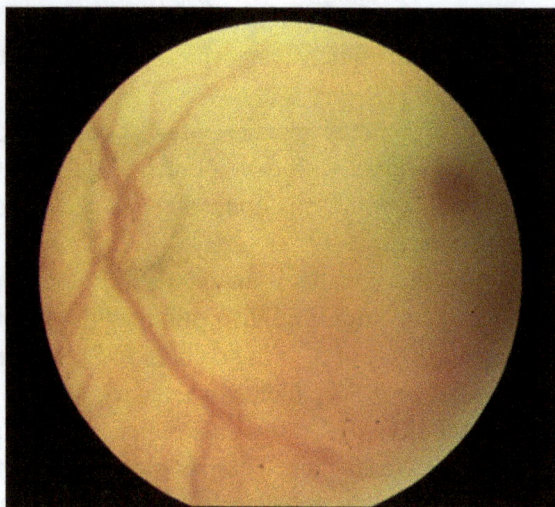

Figure 2.2. Cherry-red spot: red macula surrounded by a pale retina, reflecting the storage material in the perifoveal ganglion cells.

Table 2.5. Disorders associated with the cherry-red spot and additional features.

• Galactosialidosis	Cerebellar ataxia, myoclonus, visual failure; onset in late childhood or adolescence
• G_{M1}-gangliosidosis	Coarse facial features, corneal clouding, hepatomegaly, skeletal dysplasia, learning disability, myoclonus
• Infantile free sialic acid storage disease (ISSD)	Coarse facies, fair complexion, hepatosplenomegaly, and severe psychomotor retardation, nephrotic syndrome
• Mucolipidosis II (I-cell disease)	Coarse facies, short stature, kyphoscoliosis, umbilical and inguinal hernias
• Mucopolysaccharidosis types IVB and VII	Short stature, skeletal dysplasia
• Neuronal ceroid lipofuscinosis (NCL)	Cerebellar ataxia, myoclonus, visual failure; onset by late childhood or adolescence
• Niemann-Pick disease type A	Hepatosplenomegaly, spasticity
• Sialidosis type I	Juvenile or adult onset; intention and action myoclonus
• Sandhoff disease	Exaggerated acousticomotor reflex, splenomegaly
• Tay-Sachs disease	Exaggerated acousticomotor reflex, megalencephaly

common problem in adult patients with *AFD*. Abnormalities of brainstem auditory evoked response can be seen in *neuronopathic Gaucher disease, metachromatic leukodystrophy (MLD)* and *Krabbe disease*.

Neurologic problems (Table 2.2)

Leukodystrophy is found in *Krabbe disease* and *MLD*, associated with spasticity. Signs of peripheral neuropathy are also usually noted in these patients. White matter signal abnormalities (leukoariosis) noted on brain imaging can be encountered in adults with *AFD*, in the absence of gross cognitive deficits.[9] Cerebrovascular involvement in *AFD* can lead to transient ischemic attacks or stroke. The presence of acroparesthesis, sweating abnormalities and cardiac conduction abnormalities and pro-teinuria are additional features of *AFD*.

Progressive developmental decline or regression occurs in the *sphingolipidoses* and severe variants of the *MPS* and *oligosaccharidoses*. Associated behavioral problems are seen in the *MPS*; interestingly, those with *MPS type I* disease tend to be placid initially, whereas children with either *MPS type II* or *III* are hyperactive and can be aggressive before ultimately showing a decline.[10] Somatic features of disease (e.g., coarse facies and hepatosplenomegaly), which are characteristically noted in children with *MPS-I* and *II,* tend to be subtle in children with *MPS-III*. Hearing deficits may be a factor which contributes to developmental delay or decline in patients with *MPS*.

Arrested neurologic development and visual impairment are presenting features in patients with *NCL* and *ML-IV*.[11,12] Myoclonic seizures and pyramidal and extra-pyramidal motor dysfunction point to the *NCLs*; a heterogeneous group of neurodegenerative disorders divided into individual subtypes on the basis of age at onset: congenital, late-infantile-, juvenile- and adult-onset (Kuf's) disease. In *ML-IV*, motor problems usually begin between 3 and 8 months of age, and most patients eventually lose the ability to walk independently; speech is also generally lacking. Dysmorphic facial features or skeletal abnormalities do not occur in either *NCL* or *ML-IV*, which are characterized by eye findings that can support the clinical diagnosis in suspected cases.

Ataxia with cerebellar atrophy is a prominent sign in the later-onset forms of G_{M2}-*gangliosidosis*, associated with proximal weakness as a consequence of anterior motor horn involvement. Ataxia may also develop in patients with *Gaucher disease (GD type III)*, in whom oculomotor apraxia, hepatosplenomegaly and bone disease can be found. Other disorders associated with ataxia include *Niemann-Pick type C (NPC), late-infantile and juvenile Krabbe disease, α-mannosidosis, galactosialidosis, NCL,* and *Salla disease.*[13] Features that are distinctive for *galactosialidosis* include the presence of a cherry-red macular spot, dysmorphic facial features, hepatomegaly and skeletal changes.

Seizures are common in several LSDs, but usually develop later or during advanced stages of the disease process, except in *NCL* and *GD type III.*[14] In *late-infantile NCL (LINCL),* symptoms usually appear in young children between the ages of 2 and 4 years.[11] Affected children develop myoclonus and loss of motor function and language, and by the age of 6 years, the children are usually unable to walk and sit unsupported and become blind. Death in these cases typically occurs in mid-childhood.

Behavioral abnormalities, cognitive deficits and dementia may be the initial presentation in a patient with a *late-onset form of MLD* or *Tay-Sachs disease (TSD).*[15] Eventually these patients develop a progressive disorder of gait or coordination, and a progressive polyneuropathy. Neuropsychological assessment in patients with *late-onset MLD* has demonstrated the presence of mild amnesia, visuo-spatial dysfunction and attention deficits, and a slow psychomotor speed. Cerebellar atrophy on brain MRI is seen in patients with *late-onset TSD,* whereas patients with *MLD* have signal abnormalities that are consistent with a demyelinating form of leukodystrophy.

A majority of patients with *MPS-IIIA* first present with behavioral abnormalities and sleep disturbances in the first year of life.[16] Dementia also becomes apparent in the majority of these patients by the age of 6 years, whereas adult-onset of dementia has been reported in *MPS-IIIB* patients. Evaluations of children with non-specific developmental delay, behavioral abnormalities, or a delay in speech development should include testing for excess urinary glycosaminoglycans and oligosaccharides. Elevated oligosaccharide levels are observed in the *glycoproteinoses,* such as *fucosidosis* and *aspartylglycosaminuria;* disorders associated with behavioral and speech problems. Children with *aspartylglycosaminuria* display alternating periods of hyperactivity and apathy.[3]

Peripheral neuropathy caused by a disruption in the integrity of peripheral myelin can be found in *MLD* and *Krabbe disease*, associated with varying degrees of abnormalities on testing of visual, brainstem auditory and somatosensory evoked potential. In the *MPS*, carpal tunnel syndrome may develop as a result of median nerve compression. Manual dexterity can be further compromised in children with *MPS*, as a consequence of the underlying skeletal dysplasia and associated 'claw hand deformity'.

Sensory-motor polyneuropathy has been described in an adult patient with *Schindler/Kanzaki disease* (*α-N-acetylgalactosaminidase deficiency*); sural nerve biopsy has revealed decreased density of myelinated fibers and axonal degeneration.[17]

Myopathy is a feature of *Pompe* and *Danon disease*, both of which are associated with cardiomyopathy.[18,19] Patients with the later-onset form of *Pompe disease* (*acid maltase myopathy*) and *Danon disease* manifest with progressive proximal myopathy and gait problems, often mistakenly attributed to limb girdle muscular dystrophy. Gait problems are also seen in patients with *MPS* disorders, but this is attributed to the underlying skeletal dysplasia and joint contractures. However, spinal cord compression, due to pachymeningitis, can develop in patients with *MPS*, which can manifest as motor deficits.[20] In addition, patients with *MPS* and odontoid hypoplasia may develop myelopathy with cervical subluxation.

Cardiopulmonary problems

Pulmonary involvement is a characteristic feature of several LSDs. Recurrent and persistent upper respiratory tract infections, with chronic rhinorrhea and otitis media, are early problems in children with *MPS*.[21] Eventually these patients develop obstructive upper airway symptoms due to tracheal narrowing, and enlargement of the tonsils and adenoids from GAGs accumulation. Sleep apnea is also common in these patients.[22]

Obstructive airway disease may contribute to limitations in exercise tolerance among patients with *AFD*, in whom cardiac-related complications are also common.

Interstitial lung disease has been described in patients with *GD type III* and *Niemann-Pick disease*.

Cardiac involvement in *AFD* and the *MPS* disorders can manifest with cardiac hypertrophy and valvular disease. In *AFD*, most patients also experience arrhythmias and develop a block in cardiac conduction. Similar problems are encountered in *Danon disease*. Additional features that are distinctive for *Danon disease* include mental retardation (70% of male cases) and myopathy.[23] Valvular heart disease is common among patients with *MPS*. Cardiomyopathy is not encountered in the late-onset form of Pompe disease; but affected individuals are at risk for respiratory failure.

Visceral problems

Hepatosplenomegaly is encountered primarily in LSDs associated with infiltration of the bone marrow and reticulo-endothelial system, such as *GD, Niemann-Pick disease, MPS* and *oligosaccharidoses*. However, hepatic synthetic function in these patients is usually intact; although markedly enlarged spleens may lead to hypersplenism and a low platelet count.

Deposition of sulfatides in the gallbladder of patients with *MLD* can cause the formation of papillomatous changes and lead to cholecystitis. Gallstones and cholecystitis have also been reported among adult patients with *GD*.

Renal dysfunction can develop in *cystinosis* and *Anderson-Fabry disease*. In the early-onset form of *cystinosis*, there is proximal tubular dysfunction leading to glucosuria and proteinuria (Fanconi syndrome), starting from the age of 6–12 months.[24] Associated features include growth retardation, rickets and photophobia; the latter due to cystine crystal deposition in the cornea. Untreated patients develop end-stage renal disease by the age of 10 years. There is a later-onset form of *cystinosis* which can lead to renal failure in early adulthood, unless treatment is initiated. There is also a benign, non-nephropathic variant in which the phenotype is restricted to crystal deposits in the cornea and bone marrow.

In *Anderson-Fabry disease*, renal involvement may initially manifest as proteinuria and isosthenuria; evolving to chronic renal insufficiency and renal failure, usually between ages 35 and 45 years.[25] Acroparesthesias and

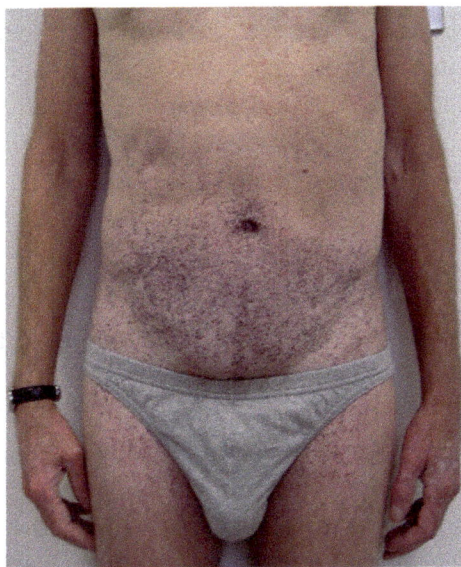

Figure 2.3. Angiokeratomas in a patient with *Anderson-Fabry disease*. Note the bathing trunk distribution.

the presence of angiokeratomas (Figure 2.3) are early findings, usually noted before age 10 in males and later among symptomatic females.[26] The presence of corneal opacities, detected by slit lamp examination, is a valuable diagnostic clue in this context.

Skeletal problems

Bone complications can be a source of debility in patients with an LSD, such as *GD* and the *MPS*.[27] In patients with *GD*, bone infarcts can provoke a bone crisis; an episode of intense bone pain, often involving the lower extremity, which is often associated with erythema and tenderness over the affected area. Progressive marrow infiltration and osteoclast activation in *GD* can lead to osteopenia and osteonecrosis of the femoral or humeral head. Osteopenia has also been described in patients with *Anderson-Fabry* and *Pompe disease*.

In the *MPS* disorders, the combination of skeletal dysplasia and joint contractures lead to stunting of growth, limitations in joint range of motion and gait problems. The spectrum of skeletal findings (dysostosis multiplex) seen in these patients is evident radiographically as gibbus deformity, and varus and valgus deformity of the feet. Similar findings, although they can be subtle, are evident in the *oligosaccharidoses*, *sialdosis type II (mucolipidosis I)* and *galactosialidosis*.

Summary

The LSDs are multi-systemic disorders characterized by wide hetero-geneity in clinical presentation. Any combination of clinical problems, which may manifest at any age may turn out to be an LSD, particularly when persistent or progressive and not readily explained. Information regarding family history may provide an important clue. Once a diagnosis of an LSD is established, it is important to perform a comprehensive assessment so that disease burden can be clarified (see Chapter 4), and a comprehensive treatment plan can be put into effect (Chapter 6).

References

1. Wilcox WR. Lysosomal storage disorders: The need for better pediatric recognition and comprehensive care. *J Pediatr.* 2004 May;144(5 Suppl.):S3–S14.
2. Kooper AJ, Janssens PM, de Groot AN, Liebrand-van Sambeek ML, van den Berg CJ, Tan-Sindhunata GB, van den Berg PP, Bijlsma EK, Smits AP, Wevers RA. Lysosomal storage diseases in non-immune hydrops fetalis pregnancies. *Clin Chim Acta.* 2006;371(1–2):176–182.
3. Arvio P, Arvio M. Progressive nature of aspartylglucosaminuria. *Acta Paediatr.* 2002;91(3):255–257.
4. Al Sawaf S, Mayatepek E, Hoffmann B. Neurological findings in Hunter disease: Pathology and possible therapeutic effects reviewed. *J Inherit Metab Dis.* 2008;31(4):473–480.
5. Torvin Møller A, Staehelin Jensen T. Neurology in Fabry disease. *Clin Ther.* 2008;30(Suppl. B):S47–S49.
6. Prall FR, Drack A, Taylor M, *et al.* Ophthalmic manifestations of Danon disease. *Ophthalmology.* 2006;113:1010–1013.

7. Ganguly S, Gabani RU, Chakraborty S, Ganguly SB. Sialidosis type I (cherry-red spot-myoclonus syndrome). *J Indian Med Assoc.* 2004 March;102(3):174–175.

8. Leavitt JA, Kotagal S. The "cherry red" spot. *Pediatr Neurol.* 2007;37(1): 74–75.

9. Fellgiebel A, Keller I, Marin D, Müller MJ, Schermuly I, Yakushev I, Albrecht J, Bellhäuser H, Kinateder M, Beck M, Stoeter P. Diagnostic utility of different MRI and MR angiography measures in Fabry disease. *Neurology.* 2009;72(1):63–68.

10. Bax MC, Colville GA. Behaviour in mucopolysaccharide disorders. *Arch Dis Child.* 1995;73(1):77–81.

11. Jalanko A, Braulke T. Neuronal ceroid lipofuscinoses. *Biochim Biophys Acta.* 2009;1793(4):697–709.

12. Altarescu G, Sun M, Moore DF, Smith JA, Wiggs EA, Solomon BI, Patronas NJ, Frei KP, Gupta S, Kaneski CR, Quarrell OW, Slaugenhaupt SA, Goldin E, Schiffmann R. The neurogenetics of mucolipidosis type IV. *Neurology.* 2002;59(3):306–313.

13. Parker CC, Evans OB. Metabolic disorders causing childhood ataxia. *Semin Pediatr Neurol.* 2003;10(3):193–199.

14. Sedel F, Gourfinkel-An I, Lyon-Caen O, Baulac M, Saudubray JM, Navarro V. Epilepsy and inborn errors of metabolism in adults: a diagnostic approach. *J Inherit Metab Dis.* 2007;30(6):846–854.

15. Sedel F, Baumann N, Turpin JC, Lyon-Caen O, Saudubray JM, Cohen D. Psychiatric manifestations revealing inborn errors of metabolism in adolescents and adults. *J Inherit Metab Dis.* 2007;30(5):631–641.

16. Valstar MJ, Ruijter GJ, van Diggelen OP, Poorthuis BJ, Wijburg FA. Sanfilippo syndrome: a mini-review. *J Inherit Metab Dis.* 2008 April 4.

17. Kodama K, Kobayashi H, Abe R, Ohkawara A, Yoshii N, Yotsumoto S, Fukushige T, Nagatsuka Y, Hirabayashi Y, Kanzaki T. A new case of alpha-N-acetylgalactosaminidase deficiency with angiokeratoma corporis diffusum, with Ménière's syndrome and without mental retardation. *Br J Dermatol.* 2001;144(2):363–368.

18. Van der Beek NA, Hagemans ML, Reuser AJ, Hop WC, Van der Ploeg AT, Van Doorn PA, Wokke JH. Rate of disease progression during long-term follow-up of patients with late-onset Pompe disease. *Neuromuscul Disord.* 2009;19(2):113–117.

19. Sugie K, Yamamoto A, Murayama K, Oh SJ, Takahashi M, Mora M, Riggs JE, Colomer J, Iturriaga C, Meloni A, Lamperti C, Saitoh S, Byrne E, DiMauro S, Nonaka I, Hirano M, Nishino I. Clinicopathological features of genetically confirmed Danon disease. *Neurology.* 2002;58(12):1773–1778.

20. Boor R, Miebach E, Brühl K, Beck M. Abnormal somatosensory evoked potentials indicate compressive cervical myelopathy in mucopolysaccharidoses. *Neuropediatrics.* 2000;31(3):122–127.

21. Kamin W. Diagnosis and management of respiratory involvement in Hunter syndrome. *Acta Paediatr Suppl.* 2008;97(457):57–60.

22. Yeung AH, Cowan MJ, Horn B, Rosbe KW. Airway management in children with mucopolysaccharidoses. *Arch Otolaryngol Head Neck Surg.* 2009; 135(1):73–79.

23. Sugie K, Yamamoto A, Murayama K, Oh SJ, Takahashi M, Mora M, Riggs JE, Colomer J, Iturriaga C, Meloni A, Lamperti C, Saitoh S, Byrne E, DiMauro S, Nonaka I, Hirano M, Nishino I. Clinicopathological features of genetically confirmed Danon disease. *Neurology.* 2002;58(12):1773–1778.

24. Nesterova G, Gahl W. Nephropathic cystinosis: late complications of a multisystemic disease. *Pediatr Nephrol.* 2008;23(6):863–878.

25. Torra R. Renal manifestations in Fabry disease and therapeutic options. *Kidney Int Suppl.* 2008;(111):S29–S32.

26. Ramaswami U. Fabry disease during childhood: clinical manifestations and treatment with agalsidase alfa. *Acta Paediatr Suppl.* 2008;97(457):38–40.

27. Pastores GM. Musculoskeletal complications encountered in the lysosomal storage disorders. *Best Pract Res Clin Rheumatol.* 2008;22(5):937–947.

Vignette

JC had normal development up to age of 14 months, when he displayed difficulties in standing and walking (attributed to hypotonia). He was seen by a neurologist, and had testing of motor nerve conduction velocity which indicated a demyelinating peripheral polyneuropathy. Subsequently, he developed spasticity with brisk tendon reflexes; brain MRI revealed the presence of a leukodystrophy. *Metachromatic leukodystrophy (MLD)* or *Krabbe disease* were entertained as possible diagnoses. Tests revealed decreased arylsulfatase A (ARSA) activity and the presence of urine sulfatides; these findings were deemed confirmatory of the diagnosis of *MLD*. Mutation analyses were performed and revealed a novel ARSA gene sequence alteration, W193C (TGG579TGT), inherited from the mother. In addition, the maternal allele was also found to have the N350S (AAT1424AGT) mutation, which is associated with pseudo-deficient ARSA activity. Sequence analysis did not show an ARSA mutation on the paternal allele, although an ARSA gene polymorphism was identified; this information was deemed potentially useful in identifying the disease-carrying paternal allele.

During a second pregnancy the mother requested prenatal testing, which revealed that the fetus had decreased ARSA activity. In addition, mutation analyses revealed test results consistent with that found in the affected sibling. However, there was concern about the low but detectable ARSA activity, which in this case was found to be above the laboratory's usual range of values seen in classically affected *MLD* patients. This finding raised the possibility of an alternative diagnosis, *multiple sulfatase (MSD) deficiency*. Analysis of the MSD gene (*SUMF1*) in the index patient (JC) revealed the presence of two previously described mutations; indicating compound heterozygosity (A279V/C218Y). These results helped to establish the correct diagnosis (*MSD*) as the basis for JC's clinical problems. Testing of the current pregnancy revealed the fetus was a carrier, but not affected by *MSD* and the low ARSA activity was attributed to the presence of the pseudo-deficiency allele.

SUMF1 encodes a protein involved in the post-translational modification of several sulfatases. Deficient activity of individual sulfatases, such as of ARSA and iduronate-2-sulfatase (I2S), can lead to distinct LSDs; specifically *MLD* and *Hunter syndrome*, respectively. Measuring the activity of two or more sulfates is required, when these diagnoses are suspected, to ensure that a diagnosis of *MSD* is not missed. With regards to ARSA activity, the presence of a pseudo-deficiency can lead to an erroneous diagnosis of *MLD*. Additionally, rare patients with saposin B (Sap-B) deficiency have been described, with clinical features that overlap with a *juvenile-onset form of MLD*. Sap-B acts as an activator of ARSA and is required for the hydrolysis of galactosylsulfatide. In patients with deficient ARSA activity the presence of excess sulfatides in urine is supportive evidence of an *in vivo* deficiency in enzyme activity. Mutation analysis can complement the results obtained with biochemical testing. However, one must be cautious in interpreting the significance of gene sequence alterations, particularly when such alterations are not previously described in other affected families. Causality is often demonstrated on the basis of mutagenesis and protein expression studies. As evident in the case described, the diagnosis of an LSD can be confounded by several factors, and consultation with experts in the field may help prevent misdiagnosis or the introduction of inappropriate treatment.

Suggested Reading

Biffi A, Lucchini G, Rovelli A, Sessa M. Metachromatic leukodystrophy: an overview of current and prospective treatments. *Bone Marrow Transplant.* 2008;42(Suppl. 2):S2–S6.

Deconinck N, Messaaoui A, Ziereisen F, Kadhim H, Sznajer Y, Pelc K, Nassogne MC, Vanier MT, Dan B. Metachromatic leukodystrophy without arylsulfatase

A deficiency: a new case of saposin-B deficiency. *Eur J Paediatr Neurol.* 2008;12(1):46–50.

Dierks T, Schlotawa L, Frese MA, Radhakrishnan K, von Figura K, Schmidt B. Molecular basis of multiple sulfatase deficiency, mucolipidosis II/III and Niemann-Pick C1 disease — Lysosomal storage disorders caused by defects of non-lysosomal proteins. *Biochim Biophys Acta.* 2009;1793(4):710–725.

3

Diagnostic Confirmation and Screening Protocols

The LSDs are hereditary diseases, transmitted mainly as autosomal recessive traits, except for the following X-linked disorders: *Anderson-Fabry disease (AFD), Hunter syndrome (MPS-II)* and *Danon disease.* Biochemical testing is available for most LSDs, enabling diagnostic confirmation in suspected clinical cases, and prenatal diagnosis can also be offered to carrier couples at risk of having an affected child. Carrier detection is available, primarily by molecular assays for particular disorders in defined populations at high risk, and among relatives of an affected individual whose gene defects have been identified.

The availability of confirmatory testing through blood tests should obviate the need for invasive procedures, such as bone marrow, skin or liver biopsy. In the past and particularly in locations where there are no laboratories with the requisite expertise, biopsies were often done to establish the presence of tissue deposits, which served as a presumptive basis for diagnosis of an LSD. Examination of blood films for evidence of vacuolated lymphocytes in suspected cases is a simple test; this finding has been described in several LSDs (Figure 3.1; Table 3.1).[1] Subsequently, the diagnosis can be confirmed by appropriate biochemical or molecular assays.

Although individual entities are rare, collectively the estimated incidence of the LSDs is about 1 in 5,000 live births. Some conditions are known to be prevalent in certain ethnic groups, on account of founder effect, the phenomenon of shared identity by descent (i.e., blood lines). For instance, among Ashkenazi Jews (AJ), the relative incidence of

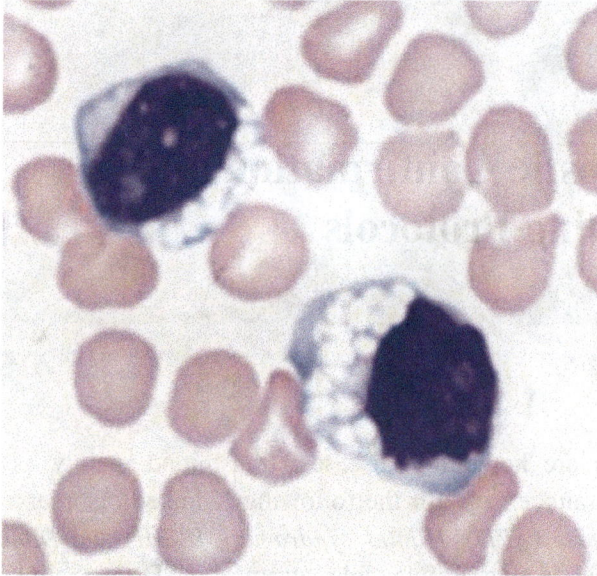

Figure 3.1. Vacuolated lymphocyte.

Table 3.1. Diseases associated with abnormal cytoplasmic vacuolation of lymphocytes.

- Batten's disease (neuronal ceroid lipofuscinosis)
- Fucosidosis
- G_{M1}-gangliosidosis (β-galactosidase deficiency)
- Galactosialidosis
- I-cell disease (mucolipidosis II)
- Mannosidosis
- Mucopolysaccharidoses
- Neuraminidase/sialidase deficiency
- Niemann-Pick disease
- Pompe disease (glycogenosis Type II)
- Salla disease
- Wolman's disease

---

mucolipidosis IV and a subset of the sphingolipidoses (i.e., *Gaucher disease, Tays-Sachs and Niemann Pick type A*) is higher, compared with other groups (Table 3.2).[2] Within the AJ community, the introduction of screening programs prior to marriage introductions among the Orthodox

Table 3.2. Diseases prevalent among the Ashkenazi and the commonly found mutations.*

Disease	Common Mutations	Carrier Frequency
Gaucher	5: N370S; 84GG; L444P; IVS2^{+1}; R496H;	1:16
Tay-Sachs Disease	3: 4-BP ins, EX11; IVS12	1:27
Mucolipidosis type IV	2: c.416-2A>G; c.1_788del	1:98
Niemann Pick type A/B	3: R496L; L302P; fs330	1:110

*Bach G, Zeigler M, Zlotogora J. Prevention of lysosomal storage disorders in Israel. *Mol Genet Metab.* 2007;90(4):353–357.

community, and screening in other groups to identify couples at risk (so they may be offered prenatal diagnosis), has drastically reduced the number of affected cases.

In the past few years, and especially following the introduction of enzyme replacement therapy for several LSDs, specialized centers for the diagnosis and care of affected individuals have been established. This is an ideal situation, as the complex medical and psychosocial issues confronting patients with LSDs often require management by a multidisciplinary team. Several disease-specific registries or observational surveys have also been established to facilitate characterization of disease course and substantiate the efficacy of treatment.

Diagnostic confirmation, including prenatal diagnosis

Biochemical and molecular assays can be conducted to diagnose an LSD, using a variety of clinical material, such as plasma, leukocytes or cultured fibroblasts, and urine. In cases where prenatal diagnosis is required, cultured CVS or amniocytes can be used for analysis.

Testing is available only through specialized laboratories, which means that most clinicians will have to ship the sample obtained from a patient suspected to have an LSD to a referral facility. As improper handling can affect the results of assays to measure enzyme activity, it is important to check the type and amount of clinical material required, and the proper tubes/flasks for sample collection and shipping, etc. For instance, serum and plasma are not suitable for enzymatic diagnosis of *fucosidosis* as a proportion of individuals in the general population who are otherwise healthy may have markedly decreased enzymatic activity in these body fluids. Prior to development of assays involving blood samples on filter paper, enzyme assays necessitated whole blood obtained from the patient in heparinized 'green top' tubes, while mutation detection required DNA isolation from whole blood in EDTA 'lavender top' tubes. Currently, techniques have been developed, using blood samples obtained from Guthrie cards; however, this method of testing remains the subject of on-going validation.[3]

The wide availability of biochemical and molecular assays has obviated the need to examine tissue, such as skin, bone marrow or liver.[4] Besides, histological analysis is an expensive and invasive means of pursuing diagnosis, which requires expertise that is now not generally available. The characteristic tissue findings found in various LSDs are noted in Chapter 5.

Biochemical Testing

Analysis of enzyme activity is generally performed using an artificial fluorescent tag, such as 4-methylumbelliferone, which is linked to an analog of the appropriate substrate via the relevant bond. For certain conditions, it may be necessary to use the natural substrate, which is radioactively labeled.

The enzyme assays are usually run with a known affected, unaffected and carrier individual for reference, when appropriate samples are available. In most cases, it is useful to have results not only for the enzyme whose deficiency is suspected, but also the activity of a second enzyme whose activity is expected to be normal, which serves as an internal control, particularly when the analysis is done on a shipped sample. Testing of the parents is ideal, as these results may provide a fuller picture and can clarify the situation, especially in cases wherein a pseudo-deficiency may exist. As carriers have residual enzyme activity that may overlap with the general population, biochemical assays are not ideal for assignment of carrier status. In any case, the results of testing have to be correlated with the clinical context.

Points of note

In *MLD* (arylsulfatase A deficiency), the presence of a pseudo-deficiency allele can confound assignment of true status, which may be clarified by mutation analysis. Individuals with *MLD* have excess urinary sulfatide excretion. In individuals shown to have arylsulfatase A deficiency, it is important to check the activity of other sulfatases, to exclude the diagnosis of *multiple sulfatase deficiency (MSD)*.

In patients with an *MLD-like phenotype with normal arylsulfatase A activity in vitro*, consideration should be given to the remote possibility of saposin B (Sap-B) deficiency.[5]

In patients suspected to have *Gaucher disease* (glucocerebrosidase deficiency) with typical storage cells in bone marrow but normal enzyme activity *in vitro*, consideration should be given to the remote possibility of saposin C (Sap-C) deficiency. Sap-C is required for *in vivo* hydrolysis of glucocerebroside. Patients with *Sap-C deficiency* have been described to have features consistent with *GD*, with and without neuronopathic features.[6] Recently, patients with a *LIMP1* defect, progressive myoclonic epilepsy and nephrotic syndrome have been described.[7] Testing in one of these patients revealed normal glucocerebrosidase activity in leukocytes, but a severe enzymatic deficiency in cultured skin fibroblasts. LIMP1 is required for the intralysosomal delivery of newly synthesized glucocerebrosidase, unlike most of the other lysosomal enzymes that are targeted to the lysosome via the mannose-6-phosphate receptor.

Testing for *Pompe disease* using leukocytes or lymphocytes involves the measurement of α-glucosidase activity after acarbose inhibition to neutralize non-lysosomal enzyme activity.[8]

In patients suspected to have an *MPS* disorder, the presence of excess urinary GAGs may be tested with the Berry 'spot test', a dye binding assay. A negative result does not exclude a probable diagnosis of *MPS*, and further testing may be necessary. Additional tests may include qualitative analysis by electrophoresis, or directly measuring the activity of the relevant enzyme. The pattern of urinary GAGs excretion may suggest the likely diagnosis (Table 3.3). Recently, patients with *MPS* have been found to have elevated serum levels of heparan co-factor II thrombin and an increase in the ratio of apolipoprotein CI' (ApoCI'):ApoCI.[9,10] The potential

Table 3.3. Pattern of urinary GAG excretion.*

Disease	Urinary GAG
MPS-I	HS, DS
MPS-II	HS, DS
MPS-III	HS
MPS-IV	CS, KS
MPS-VI	CS, DS
MPS-VII	DS

*MPS — mucopolysaccharidosis; CS — chondroitin sulfate; DS — dermatan sulfate; HS — heparan sulfate; KS — keratan sulfate.

role of these markers in the diagnosis and management of *MPS* patients remains to be defined (see Chapter 5).

In patients suspected to have an *oligosaccharidoses*, the urine can be checked for oligosaccharides by thin layer chromatography (TLC) followed by orcinol spray. Oligosaccharides are present in glycoproteins (covalently attached to a peptide backbone), and require extraction from biologic matrices including GAGs prior to quantitation. Urine oligosaccharides is found to be elevated in *aspartylglucosaminuria, mucolipidosis II/III, G_{M1}-gangliosidosis, Sandhoff disease, fucosidosis, α-mannosidosis, sialidosis, galactosialidosis, sialic acid storage disease* and *sialuria* (a non-LSD caused by mutations in the allosteric site of UDP-N-acetylglucosamine-2-epimerase). Free sialic acid is detected with resorcinol spray (instead of orcinol) following TLC, and also by either spectrophotometric or fluorometric thiobarbituric acid assay.

Molecular Testing

Analysis which leads to characterization of the causal gene defect(s) may provide additional information to corroborate the results of biochemical testing. Mutation detection is also a more reliable means of carrier detection, as carriers often have a biochemical assay result that falls within the range obtained for the general population. In disorders which are caused by defects in a non-lysosomal enzyme (e.g., activator, membrane or transport protein), analysis of the relevant gene sequence may be the only available means to establish a diagnosis. For families at risk of having an affected child, knowledge of the gene defects in the index patient may permit pre-implantation and/or prenatal diagnosis.

Common mutations are present for a number of LSDs, particularly for defined populations; obviating the need to sequence the entire gene in some cases:

- Among individuals of Ashkenazi Jewish descent, there are several common mutations in LSDs prevalent in this community (Table 3.2).[11] For *TSD*, the G269S mutation has been associated with a late-onset form of the disease.
- In *juvenile NCL* (*Batten disease*) a 1.02 kb deletion (c.462-677del) accounts for 85% of disease alleles in patients of European extraction.[12]
- Among patients of northern European descent with *cystinosis*, a common 57 kb deletion accounts for ~50% of disease alleles.[13]
- The majority (95%) of Finnish patients with *Salla disease* have a missense mutation (R39C) in the gene for sialin.[14] *Aspartylglycosaminuria*, also a common LSD among Finns (carrier frequency 1:30), is attributed to one common mutation identified as AGUFinn major.[14]
- A deletion mutation (502del) in the β-GALC gene has been reported as common, accounting for up to 40% of *Krabbe disease* alleles. Homozygosity for this mutation is associated with the severe *infantile* form of the disease. Mutation analysis in patient with *late-onset* disease often reveals compound heterozygosity; the 809G>A (G270D) and 1609G > A (G537R) mutations are among the alleles identified.[15]
- Two gene defects, namely 459[+1] G to A and 1277 C to T (Pro426Leu), account for almost 50% of *MLD*-causing mutations.[16] In a study of 12 cases of adult *MLD*, patients with primary motor signs (pyramidal and cerebellar signs, and less often dystonia) and peripheral neuropathy had the major adult *ARSA* mutation P426L in homozygosity.[17] In contrast, patients with the psycho-cognitive forms (associated with modifications of mood, peculiar social reactions and a progressive mental deterioration) were often noted to be compound heterozygotes, with the I179S mutation on one allele.[17] In a separate study, screening for mutations in 34 unrelated *MLD* patients from Poland

revealed that the I179S mutation accounted for 17% of examined alleles (2/12) in adults, and as much as 42% (5/12 alleles) in *late juvenile MLD* patients.[18] The I179S mutation has not been found in the *late infantile* nor in *early juvenile* cases.

Polymorphisms (i.e., two AG transitions at nucleotides 1788 and 2723) that give rise to ARSA-pseudodeficiency are common in the general population (~10%).

- Most European patients (up to 70%) with adult-onset *Pompe disease* share the same gene defect; namely, a splicing out of exon 2 caused by a 13 T to G transversion in intron 1.[19]

Information on common mutant alleles in defined populations may facilitate diagnosis and screening. Issues relating to genetic testing are best handled by referral to a medical geneticist (see below).

Specialized Testing and Other Considerations

The diagnosis of non-enzymatic defects causing LSDs requires specialized techniques that may only be available in a limited number of laboratories. Analysis of lipid profile and pattern of urine substrate excretion by tandem mass spectrometry is one of several methods being examined, as a means of rapid diagnosis.

- In *Niemann-Pick type C*, diagnosis is established by showing a defect in cholesterol esterification and/or filipin staining, both of which requires cultured skin fibroblasts (Figure 3.2). At least two different genes (NPC1 and 2) are involved, although the majority (>95%) of cases result from defects of NPC1.[20] Thus, molecular testing is done preferably after the biochemical diagnosis is ascertained.
- Patients with *multiple sulfatase deficiency* (*MSD*) and *mucolipidosis II/III* (*ML*) show abnormalities in the activity of several lysosomal enzyme, when measured in plasma (*ML*) or leukocytes (*MSD*).[21]
- In *galactosialidosis*, deficient levels of β-galactosidase and neuraminidase activity can be found, although β-galactosidase levels can be significant when measured in cultured skin fibroblasts.[22]

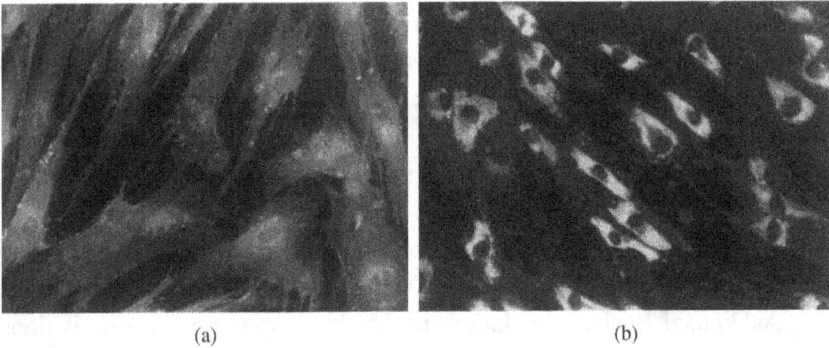

Figure 3.2. Filipin-stained cultured fibroblast: (a) normal control, (b) patients with *NPC*. The increased fluorescence intensity reflects the vacuolar accumulation of unesterified cholesterol in the perinuclear region of the NPC cells.

- The biochemical diagnosis of activator protein deficiencies requires a combination of approaches, including examination of substrate in urine (e.g., sulfatide in *Sap-B deficiency* and glucocerebroside in *Sap-C deficiency*).[23] Alternatively, the rate of radiolabeled substrate turnover in cultured skin fibroblasts can be measured through substrate loading tests. Mutation analysis can also be performed.

- The absence of LAMP2 protein on staining of skeletal muscle is a way to establish the diagnosis of *Danon disease.*[13]

- *Cystinosis* can be diagnosed, based on determination of intracellular cystine levels in polymorphonuclear leukocytes (neutrophils) or by examining the uptake of ^{35}S-cysteine into cultured fibroblasts.[13]

- In *sialic acid storage disorders (SASD)*, there is increased amounts of free sialic acid in serum and urine, which can be quantified by high-performance liquid chromatography-tandem mass spectrometry.[24] *SASD* can be distinguished from sialuria by subcellular fractionation of culured fibroblast to show the site of sialic acid storage as lysosomal (in *SASD*) or cytoplasmic (sialuria).[24]

Screening Programs

Although individual conditions are infrequent to rare, and considered by regulatory agencies as 'orphan' diseases, LSDs have a combined prevalence of about 1 in 5000–8000. This relatively high occurrence has prompted investigations of the feasibility of targeted screening, including expansion of the newborn screening program as done recently within New York State for *Krabbe disease*.[25]

The rational given for such programs include:

- the high frequency of certain disorders among a defined ethnic group e.g., *Tay-Sachs, Gaucher* and *Niemann-Pick A disease* among the Ashkenazi Jewish population, in which group carrier testing is done prior to either marriage introductions among the Orthodox or the conception or birth of children among other Jewish groups;
- the potential to intervene prior to development of significant neurologic sequelae in cases that are potentially treatable when diagnosed early (e.g., hematopoietic stem cell transplantation for *Krabbe disease*), or before the onset of irreversible tissue damage, e.g., *Anderson-Fabry disease* and consideration of enzyme therapy to prevent or delay the development of renal failure or hypertrophic cardiomyopathy;
- early diagnosis also allows maximized chances for engraftment, by taking advantage of the naturally immature immune system in the neonate, combined with the reduced incidence of severe graft versus host disease when using umbilical cord blood as donor cells; and
- the opportunity for prevention by identifying at-risk families.

Methods for biochemical screening include the measurement of enzyme activity involving the elution of the enzyme from dried blood spots on a Guthrie card.[26] Alternative approaches include immune capture of the enzyme to determine protein concentration, prior to testing of its activity and measurement of substrate by-products by tandem mass spectrometry (TMS, based on *m/z* value). The potentially greater power to discriminate between affected and unaffected individuals with assays that rely on TMS suggest a substantially lower recall rate. Furthermore, TMS enables multiplexed enzyme testing.[26,27]

In defined populations and/or for disorders with a high frequency of 'common' mutations, screening by various molecular-based assays can also be undertaken. DNA extracted from dried blood spots on a Guthrie card is often done, to facilitate sample collection and shipment, if needed.

Apart from the logistical issues that will need to be addressed, practical concerns with screening programs include the identification of pre-symptomatic individuals without the ability to predict clinical severity, age of disease onset and rate of clinical progression.[28] On the other hand, identification of patients prior to onset of irreversible disease for treatable disorders offers the best opportunity for an optimal outcome.

Issues Related to Genetic Counseling

The majority of LSDs are autosomal recessive disorders; heterozygotes or carriers (that is, individuals with a single defective gene copy) often have sufficient enzyme activity generated by their other (normal) allele. In this instance, carriers do not show evidence of tissue storage or suffer from the relevant disease that segregates in their family.

There are at least three disorders, *Anderson-Fabry* and *Danon disease* and *Hunter syndrome (MPS-II)*, which are transmitted as X-linked traits. Although females who are carriers of the trait for *Hunter syndrome* do not appear to develop clinical problems related to the presence of a mutant protein, a proportion of females who are carriers of *Anderson-Fabry disease* or *Danon disease* may experience disease-related complications, which in some cases can be as severe as that found in classically affected males.[29,30] The variable expression in these carrier females has been partly attributed to lyonization (i.e., random inactivation during early embryogenesis of one of the two X-chromosomes, which results in varying proportions of the mutant gene product in different organ systems). Skewed lysonization is seen in females with an X-autosome translocation, in whom there is inactivation of the intact X chromosome. In cases wherein the X chromosome that is attached to an autosome bears a gene mutation, disease expression may be unmasked. Rare cases of females with *Hunter syndrome* have been reported in individuals who also happen to have Turner syndrome (45,X) wherein the single X chromosome that is present also bears a mutation of the gene for iduronate-2-sulfatase. Carrier testing for *Hunter syndrome* and *Anderson-Fabry disease* can be performed by examining individual hair roots (that develop from a very small number of progenitor cells), but this requires the services of a specialized laboratory and can be cumbersome. Analysis of the relevant gene sequence is now routinely done to establish female carrier status; testing in these cases can be facilitated by screening for the disease mutation initially found in an affected male relative.

Prenatal diagnosis is available for most of the LSDs, although in a majority of cases this may require the services of a specialized laboratory. Information regarding the mutation known to segregate in the family may also enable pre-implantation genetic diagnosis. In these cases, mutation analysis can be offered to relatives who may be interested in knowing their carrier status. Patients must be offered appropriate genetic counseling.

Pseudo-deficient alleles, described for the genes encoding arylsulfatase A (*MLD*), galactocerebrosidase (*Krabbe disease*), and β-glucoronidase (*Sly syndrome*) may lead to diagnostic error, particularly in the setting of prenatal diagnosis. Thus, it is important to perform appropriate testing on samples from an index case, when available. Analysis using parental cells can also provide valuable information. In all cases, prenatal diagnostic testing must exclude the possibility of maternal cell contamination.

Several disease-causing gene defects have been identified for each of the LSD subtypes; however, genotype–phenotype correlations are often imperfect. The epigenetic and environmental factors which influence or modify clinical expression remain ill-defined.

References

1. Anderson G, Smith VV, Malone M, Sebire NJ. Blood film examination for vacuolated lymphocytes in the diagnosis of metabolic disorders; retrospective experience of more than 2,500 cases from a single centre. *J Clin Pathol.* 2005;58(12):1305–1310.

2. Ostrer H. A genetic profile of contemporary Jewish populations. *Nat Rev Genet.* 2001;2(11):891–898.

3. De Jesus VR, Zhang XK, Keutzer J, Bodamer OA, Mühl A, Orsini JJ, Caggana M, Vogt RF, Hannon WH. Development and evaluation of quality control dried blood spot materials in newborn screening for lysosomal storage disorders. *Clin Chem.* 2009;55(1):158–164.

4. Alroy J, Ucci AA. Skin biopsy: a useful tool in the diagnosis of lysosomal storage diseases. *Ultrastruct Pathol.* 2006;30(6):489–503.

5. Deconinck N, Messaaoui A, Ziereisen F, Kadhim H, Sznajer Y, Pelc K, Nassogne MC, Vanier MT, Dan B. Metachromatic leukodystrophy without arylsulfatase A deficiency: a new case of saposin-B deficiency. *Eur J Paediatr Neurol.* 2008;12(1):46–50.

6. Tylki-Szymańska A, Czartoryska B, Vanier MT, Poorthuis BJ, Groener JA, Ługowska A, Millat G, Vaccaro AM, Jurkiewicz E. Non-neuronopathic Gaucher disease due to saposin C deficiency. *Clin Genet.* 2007;72(6):538–542.

7. Balreira A, Gaspar P, Caiola D, Chaves J, Beirão I, Lima JL, Azevedo JE, Miranda MC. A nonsense mutation in the LIMP-2 gene associated with progressive myoclonic epilepsy and nephrotic syndrome. *Hum Mol Genet.* 2008;17(14):2238–2243.

8. Jack RM, Gordon C, Scott CR, Kishnani PS, Bali D. The use of acarbose inhibition in the measurement of acid alpha-glucosidase activity in blood lymphocytes for the diagnosis of Pompe disease. *Genet Med.* 2006;8(5): 307–312.

9. Randall DR, Colobong KE, Hemmelgarn H, Sinclair GB, Hetty E, Thomas A, Bodamer OA, Volkmar B, Fernhoff PM, Casey R, Chan AK, Mitchell G, Stockler S, Melancon S, Rupar T, Clarke LA. Heparin cofactor II-thrombin complex: a biomarker of MPS disease. *Mol Genet Metab.* 2008;94(4):456–461.

10. Beesley CE, Young EP, Finnegan N, Jackson M, Mills K, Vellodi A, Cleary M, Winchester BG. Discovery of a new biomarker for the mucopolysaccharidoses (MPS), dipeptidyl peptidase IV (DPP-IV; CD26), by SELDI-TOF mass spectrometry. *Mol Genet Metab.* 2009;96(4):218–224.

11. Fares F, Badarneh K, Abosaleh M, Harari-Shaham A, Diukman R, David M. Carrier frequency of autosomal-recessive disorders in the Ashkenazi Jewish population: should the rationale for mutation choice for screening be reevaluated? *Prenat Diagn.* 2008;28(3):236–241.

12. Siintola E, Lehesjoki AE, Mole SE. Molecular genetics of the NCLs — Status and perspectives. *Biochim Biophys Acta.* 2006;1762(10):857–864.

13. Ruivo R, Anne C, Sagné C, Gasnier B. Molecular and cellular basis of lysosomal transmembrane protein dysfunction. *Biochim Biophys Acta.* 2009;1793(4):636–649.

14. Sipilä K, Aula P. Database for the mutations of the Finnish disease heritage. *Hum Mutat*. 2002;19(1):16–22.

15. Suzuki K. Globoid cell leukodystrophy (Krabbe's disease): update. *J Child Neurol*. 2003;18(9):595–603.

16. Biffi A, Cesani M, Fumagalli F, Del Carro U, Baldoli C, Canale S, Gerevini S, Amadio S, Falautano M, Rovelli A, Comi G, Roncarolo MG, Sessa M. Metachromatic leukodystrophy — mutation analysis provides further evidence of genotype-phenotype correlation. *Clin Genet*. 2008;74(4):349–357.

17. Baumann N, Turpin JC, Lefevre M, Colsch B. Motor and psycho-cognitive clinical types in adult metachromatic leukodystrophy: genotype/phenotype relationships? *J Physiol Paris*. 2002;96(3–4):301–306.

18. Ługowska A, Wlodarski P, Płoski R, Mierzewska H, Dudzińska M, Matheisel A, Swietochowska H, Tylki-Szymańska A. Molecular and clinical consequences of novel mutations in the arylsulfatase A gene. *Clin Genet*. 2009;75(1):57–64.

19. Kroos MA, Pomponio RJ, Hagemans ML, Keulemans JLM, Phipps M, DeRiso M, Palmer RE, Ausems MGEM, Van der Beek NAME, Van Diggelen OP, Halley DJJ, Van der Ploeg AT, Reuser AJJ. Broad Spectrum of Pompe disease in patients with the same C.-32-13T → G haplotype. *Neurology*. 2007; 68(2):110–115.

20. Runz H, Dolle D, Schlitter AM, Zschocke J. NPC-db, a Niemann-Pick type C disease gene variation database. *Hum Mutat*. 2008;29(3):345–350.

21. Dierks T, Schlotawa L, Frese MA, Radhakrishnan K, von Figura K, Schmidt B. Molecular basis of multiple sulfatase deficiency, mucolipidosis II/III and Niemann-Pick C1 disease — Lysosomal storage disorders caused by defects of non-lysosomal proteins. *Biochim Biophys Acta*. 2009;1793(4):710–725.

22. Ostrowska H, Krukowska K, Kalinowska J, Orłowska M, Lengiewicz I. Lysosomal high molecular weight multienzyme complex. *Cell Mol Biol Lett*. 2003;8(1):19–24.

23. Matsuda J, Yoneshige A, Suzuki K. The function of sphingolipids in the nervous system: lessons learnt from mouse models of specific sphingolipid activator protein deficiencies. *J Neurochem*. 2007;103(Suppl. 1):32–38.

24. Gopaul KP, Crook MA. The inborn errors of sialic acid metabolism and their laboratory investigation. *Clin Lab*. 2006;52(3–4):155–169.

25. Duffner PK, Caggana M, Orsini JJ, Wenger DA, Patterson MC, Crosley CJ, Kurtzberg J, Arnold GL, Escolar ML, Adams DJ, Andriola MR, Aron AM,

Ciafaloni E, Djukic A, Erbe RW, Galvin-Parton P, Helton LE, Kolodny EH, Kosofsky BE, Kronn DF, Kwon JM, Levy PA, Miller-Horn J, Naidich TP, Pellegrino JE, Provenzale JM, Rothman SJ, Wasserstein MP. Newborn screening for Krabbe disease: the New York state model. *Pediatr Neurol.* 2009;40(4):245–252.

26. Millington DS. Rapid and effective screening for lysosomal storage disease: how close are we? *Clin Chem.* 2008;54(10):1592–1594.

27. Zhang XK, Elbin CS, Chuang WL, Cooper SK, Marashio CA, Beauregard C, Keutzer JM. Multiplex enzyme assay screening of dried blood spots for lysosomal storage disorders by using tandem mass spectrometry. *Clin Chem.* 2008;54(10):1725–1728.

28. Fletcher JM. Screening for lysosomal storage disorders — a clinical perspective. *J Inherit Metab Dis.* 2006;29(2–3):405–408.

29. Gibas AL, Klatt R, Johnson J, Clarke JT, Katz J. Disease rarity, carrier status, and gender: a triple disadvantage for women with Fabry disease. *J Genet Couns.* 2008;17(6):528–537.

30. Maron BJ, Roberts WC, Arad M, Haas TS, Spirito P, Wright GB, Almquist AK, Baffa JM, Saul JP, Ho CY, Seidman J, Seidman CE. Clinical outcome and phenotypic expression in LAMP2 cardiomyopathy. *JAMA.* 2009;301(12):1253–1259.

Vignette

FL is a 42-year-old man who was recently diagnosed with *acid maltase myopathy (glycogen storage disease type II)*, based on demonstration of reduced acid α-glucosidase activity in peripheral blood. He had progressive walking difficulties and problems with climbing stairs, which began at age 40. His evaluations included an EMG and a muscle biopsy, which revealed the presence of glycogen-filled vacuoles. Following his diagnosis, pulmonary function tests (PFT) and a sleep study were undertaken; PFT revealed reduced vital capacity, which worsened when supine, and reduced maximal pressure readings were noted consistent with chest wall weakness. The sleep study revealed hypoventilation and changes consistent with obstructive sleep apnea, for which Bi-level PAP was recommended. The patient was placed on enzyme (myozyme) therapy, and was started on a high-protein, low-carbohydrate diet and structured physiotherapy program. Six months into his treatment program, the patient has reported increased energy level and some gains in muscle strength.

Glycogen storage disease type II (Pompe disease), in its most aggressive form, presents in infancy with hypotonia and cardiomyopathy. In the late-onset form (*acid maltase myopathy*), affected patients in their childhood or later experience progressive deterioration of muscle strength and pulmonary function. Differences in disease onset and rate of progression are partly explained by the nature of the underlying defect in the α-glucosidase gene.

A recent questionnaire-based study of 225 children and adults with *acid maltase myopathy* has revealed disease severity to be associated with disease duration and not with age. However, patients under the age of 15 included a subgroup with a more severe and rapid disease course. Death usually occurred, secondary to respiratory failure, by 6 years of age (range 0.9–24) for patients who presented before age 1 year, and by age 25 (6.5–40.5) in those who presented between 1 and 18 years of age. Mean age at death among patients who presented after 18 years was 44.9 years (25–66). Knowledge of the natural history enables appropriate counseling of affected individuals and their families.

Suggested Reading

Hagemans ML, Hop WJ, Van Doorn PA, Reuser AJ, Van der Ploeg AT. Course of disability and respiratory function in untreated late-onset Pompe disease. *Neurology.* 2006;66(4):581–583.

Kroos M, Pomponio RJ, van Vliet L, Palmer RE, Phipps M, Van der Helm R, Halley D, Reuser A; GAA Database Consortium. Update of the Pompe disease mutation database with 107 sequence variants and a format for severity rating. *Hum Mutat.* 2008;29(6):E13–26.

van der Ploeg AT, Reuser AJ. Pompe's disease. *Lancet.* 2008;372(9646): 1342–1353.

4

Assessment of Disease Burden and Assignment of Disease Severity

Evaluation of a patient with an LSD necessitates a battery of tests to ascertain the pattern and severity of disease. Serial monitoring is also required to assess current clinical status and rate of disease progression, or response to therapy. A majority of the individual clinical entities are characterized by primary central nervous system (CNS) involvement, and assignment of particular disease subtype is important for prognostication and management.

Unfortunately, only a few studies have evaluated disease burden in a quantitative fashion, and only a handful of these have systematically examined for signs of disease progression. These factors have confounded the process of identifying suitable clinical endpoints in several trials designed to assess the safety and efficacy of therapeutic interventions (see Chapter 6).

This chapter provides an overview of the various clinical investigations that are typically performed to define the specific organ/system involvement in patients diagnosed with an LSD, and the characteristic findings for a sampling of disorders. A selection of scoring systems, as a means of assigning disease severity, is also provided as a guide. Some of the tests that are described may have been undertaken during the initial evaluation of a patient for diagnostic purposes; re-evaluations may not provide additional information of use in the management of the patient. Furthermore, certain tests may only provide a qualitative or semi-quantitative description of the disease, and may lack sensitivity when used in the assessment of disease progression. Ideally, given the complex nature of disease a patient diagnosed with an LSD should be managed by a multidisciplinary team at a designated specialist center.

Nervous system involvement

Brain magnetic resonance imaging (MRI): Leukodystrophy is evident on brain MRI as symmetrical signal abnormalities in regions corresponding to brain white matter. In *Krabbe disease* this is usually noted in the periventricular region of the posterior cerebral hemispheres. In *metachromatic leukodystrophy (MLD)*, the hyperintense signal in the periventricular and central white matter on T_2-weighted images may initially be limited to the parieto-occipital region (Figure 4.1).[1]

Brain imaging in adult patients with *Anderson-Fabry disease (AFD)* often reveals the presence of white matter signal abnormalities (leukoariosis), in the absence of major cognitive impairment.[2] Additional findings include increased tortuosity of the blood vessels, predominantly in the posterior circulation (Figure 4.2). Cerebral imaging and blood flow studies in *AFD* patients, who are prone to transient ischemic attacks and

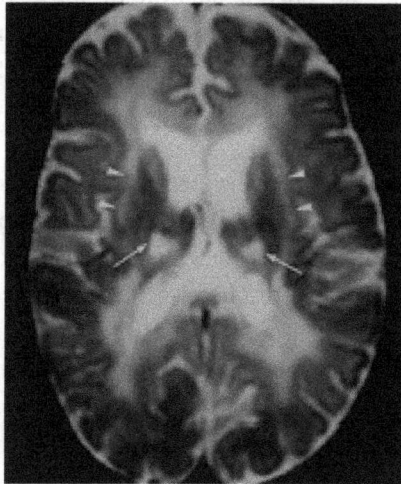

Figure 4.1. Leukodystrophy in a child with *MLD*, evident on brain MRI as changes in white matter signal in the periventricular area (arrow heads).

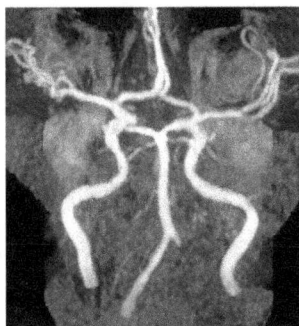

Figure 4.2. Imaging with contrast showing dilatation and tortuosity of the blood vessels in the brain posterior circulation of a patient with *Anderson-Fabry disease*.

strokes, have paradoxically shown hyperperfusion, which has been attributed to altered vascular reactivity.

MRI findings in *sialidoses* range from normal in the early stages to signs of cerebellar, pontine, and cerebral atrophy with disease progression.[3] Similar observations have been described among patients with *fucosidosis*.[4] In addition, extensive and progressive changes in the signal intensity of the white matter, involving the corpus medullare, periventricular, lobar, and subcortical supratentorial areas, internal and external capsules, and the internal medullary laminae of the thalami have been described.[4]

Serial brain imaging in patients with *late infantile NCL* demonstrates progressive gray matter atrophy (prominent in the infratentorial regions), enlarged cerebral and cerebellar sulci, as well as dilated ventricles.[5] Patients with *late-onset G_{M2}-gangliosidosis* show cerebellar atrophy.[6]

Brain MR spectroscopy (MRS) in patients with *infantile Krabbe disease* and *MLD* has revealed elevation of myo-inositol and choline (cho)-containing compounds in affected white matter, consistent with demyelination and glial proliferation.[7,8] Cho is considered as a marker of membrane destruction or gliosis, whereas *N*-acetylaspartate (NAA) is believed to reflect neuronal viability. A decrease of NAA points to neuroaxonal loss in advanced stages of the disease process.

In *Niemann-Pick type C (NPC)*, Cho/creatine (Cr) and NAA/Cr ratios were calculated in brain white matter (centrum ovale or semiovale), revealing a sustained decrease in the Cho/Cr ratio in three patients treated with miglustat.[9]

Brain MRS in patients with *Salla disease* has shown higher *N*-acetyl and phosphocreatine concentrations in parietal white matter but lower levels of Cho-containing compounds, when compared with values in age-matched controls.[10]

In *mucolipidosis type IV* (*ML-IV*), the ratios of NAA/creatine-phosphocreatine and NAA/Cho-containing compounds are significantly reduced.[11] However, no difference has been found between younger and older patients, suggesting that *ML-IV* may be a largely static developmental encephalopathy associated with diffuse neuronal and axonal damage or dysfunction.

SPECT analysis in patients with *infantile NCL* has revealed cortical hypoperfusion and loss of benzodiazepine receptors with the onset of clinical manifestations. The volume of gray matter, percentage of gray matter volume, and NAA levels decreased with age and severity of the disease; whereas ventricular volume, percentage of ventricular volume, and CADC (to assess the consequences of neuronal loss) and percentage of white matter increased.[12] In this series, the best correlations between age and the severity scales (see Table 4.5) were found with ventricular volume or percentage of ventricular volume.[12]

Brain stem auditory evoked response (ABR): Abnormalities of the ABR testing are among the first objective indications of CNS disease in patients with an LSD. Abnormal wave forms and latencies have been reported in *GD type III, Krabbe disease, MLD* and *NCL*.[13–16] It should be noted that a normal ABR test result at presentation does not necessarily exclude neuronopathic involvement, and indeed this may often be the case with later-onset or chronic forms of the disease.

Hearing tests: Conductive and/or sensorineural hearing loss have been described in patients with *MPS* disorders[17]; on the other hand patients with *Anderson-Fabry disease* suffer from high frequency hearing loss and tinnitus.[18]

Visual evoked potential (VEP): Abnormalities of VEP testing is seen in *Krabbe disease*, primarily in *early infantile* cases, *MLD*, *NCL* and

ML-IV.[14–16,19] As with ABR results, a normal VEP test result at presentation does not necessarily exclude neuronopathic involvement, particularly in later-onset or chronic forms of the disease.

Electroretinography (ERG): Patients with *ML-IV* show signs of retinal dystrophy, predominantly affecting rod and bipolar cell function.[20] ERG abnormalities have also been described in *NCL* patients.[21] In patients with *infantile NCL* ERG studies show normal scotopic bright flash a-wave amplitudes with severe loss of b-wave.

DC-electro-oculography and/or video assessments have been done to measure saccadic eye movements in *GD* and *NPC* patients. In *GD*, optokinetic and vestibular nystagmus reveals marked paucity of quick-phases making the eyes "lock up" at the limit of gaze, indicative of saccade initiation failure.[22] Patients with *NPC* have supranuclear gaze palsy; in clinical trials with miglustat, horizontal saccadic eye movement velocity was assessed and shown to improve.[23]

Cerebrospinal fluid (CSF) testing: CSF protein levels are elevated in *Krabbe disease* and *MLD*, but may only be minimally increased in late-onset forms of these diseases.[7,8]

Nerve conduction velocity (NCV): Marked reductions in conduction velocity can be seen in *Krabbe disease* and *MLD*.[15,24] Abnormal neurophysiologic studies in these patients have correlated with more extensive disease, as measured by MRI scans.[7,15,24]

Abnormalities in NCV, compatible with demyelinating polyneuropathy, have also been reported in nearly half of the patients with *Salla disease*.[25] Patients with *late-onset G_{M2}-gangliosidosis* have also been shown to have NCV abnormalities.[26]

Electromyography (EMG): Abnormalities described in *Pompe disease* include increased insertional and spontaneous activity in the form of myotonic or pseudomyotonic discharges, complex repetitive discharges, fibrillation potentials, and positive sharp waves, particularly in infantile-onset cases.[27]

Neuropsychological testing is important, and testing is best conducted at centers with expertise in the LSDs. Several LSDs can be associated with varying levels of cognitive impairment and with deficits in visual, auditory and motor systems.[28,29] Combined with assessments of adaptive function, educational programs can be devised to meet an individual child's needs.

Cardiopulmonary involvement

Pulmonary function tests (PFT): Patients with an *MPS* disorder show obstructive airway disease (decreased FEV_1), which is associated with sleep apnea.[30] A small thoracic cavity and tight chest, with an enlarged liver and spleen pushing up against the diaphragm may be noted as reductions in lung volume or capacity. The 6- and 12-minute walk test (MWT), and the 3-minute stair climb test are additional measures of cardiopulmonary function that were included in assessments of patient performance in the various *MPS* enzyme therapy trials. However, it should be noted that the underlying bone and joint disease found in patients with *MPS* are confounding factors in the assessment of overall performance during timed tests of endurance.

Respiratory muscle strength can be assessed by measuring maximal expiratory (MEP) and inspiratory (MIP) pressures. In patients with *Pompe disease*, there is diaphragmatic weakness, which is evident as a postural drop in FVC from sitting to supine of at least 10%.[31] Furthermore, children and adults with *Pompe disease* are at risk for sleep-disordered breathing (SDB), manifest as obstructive sleep apnea, REM sleep hypopneas (with or without hypoventilation), or continuous sleep hypoventilation.[31,32] SDB is evaluated by **polysomnography**.

Cardiac structure/functional tests: In classic *infantile-onset Pompe disease*, cardiomyopathy is a prominent feature; its severity can be assessed based on increase of left ventricular mass as measured by **echocardiography**.[33] **Electrocardiography** in these patients may reveal a shortening of the PR interval and tall and broad QRS complexes.[33]

Patients with *Anderson-Fabry disease* (*AFD*) are also at risk for cardiomyopathy, cardiac conduction problems and arrhythmia. Lower early diastolic tissue Doppler velocities have been described among these patients, in the presence or absence of left ventricular hypertrophy

(LVH).[34] Among patients with LVH, isovolumic relaxation time can be longer and peak systolic wall motion velocity can be lower.[34] Additionally, systolic myocardial velocity has been inversely correlated with septum and posterior wall thickness. A strong correlation between age and left ventricular mass index (LVMi, $g/m^{2.7}$) was also noted, and longitudinal follow-up has revealed an increase in LVMi by 4.07 ± 1.03 $g/m^{2.7}$ per year in males and by 2.31 ± 0.81 $g/m^{2.7}$ in females. Among those without LVH, isovolumic contraction time can be shorter.[34] Cardiac MRI with contrast may reveal areas of fibrosis. Exercise capacity, assessed by bicycle stress tests with VO_2 max measurement and the 6-MWT, can be used as an integrated measure of cardiovascular function in *AFD* patients; these tests can also be used to monitor the effects of treatment.[35] Affected individuals of the *MPS* disorders are at risk for valvular disease, cardiomyopathy, congestive heart failure and coronary artery disease.

Musculoskeletal involvement

Patients with *infantile-onset Pompe disease* exhibit hypotonia; the **Alberta Infant Motor Scale (AIMS)** score has been used as a measure of disease severity, and also in the evaluation of therapeutic response to enzyme therapy.[36]

Proximal myopathy is a feature of *late-onset Pompe disease (acid maltase deficiency)*. **Quantitative muscle testing (QMT)** has been used to measure disease burden in these patients, and found to correlate with **assessment of functional activities (FAA)**.[37] QMT entails the use of a grip dynamometer, whereas FAA involves timed testing of performance in a 10-meter walk, the 4-stair climb, and the modified Gowers' maneuver.[37]

Dysostosis multiplex, a characteristic finding in patients with *MPS* and *oligosaccharidoses*, is evident on **X-rays** as anterior beaking of the thoracolumbar spine, short bullet-shaped phalanges, and broad oar-like ribs (Figure 4.3).[38] In patients with *Gaucher disease (GD)*, X-rays reveal the presence of an Erlenmeyer flask deformity (or undertubulation of the long bone).[38] MRI with assessment of fat fraction in the lumbar spine has been used to characterize the pattern of marrow infiltration in *GD* patients, which can be monitored to provide a quantitative measure of improvement on enzyme therapy.

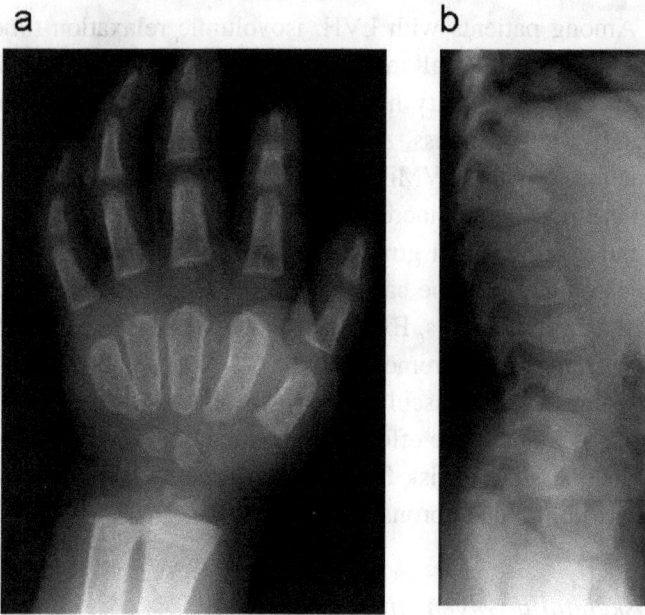

Figure 4.3. X-ray views which show (a) the bullet-shaped phalanges and (b) anterior beaking of the vertebra; consistent with dysostosis in a child with an *MPS* disorder.

Disease Severity Scores

As noted, there is a paucity of systematic studies aimed at defining the natural course of individual LSDs. Moreover, there are very few studies that have examined the correlation between disease severity and the patient's functional ability or health-related quality of life. In a few cases, a scoring system has been devised to assign disease severity. However, it has been difficult to appreciate the pattern of disease in any given patient based on a total score alone, as most clinical entities are characterized by multi-systemic involvement, and it is not unusual to find discordance in severity of individual organ/system disease.

This section provides a few examples of disease severity scoring systems for several LSDs. Potential applications include the evaluation of the role of surrogate markers, staging of the disease process (on or off treatment), stratification of patients according to disease severity to evaluate drug dose–response relationships, and facilitate communication regarding patient status among the various centers involved with their care.

Gaucher disease (*GD*). Table 4.1a: A scoring system, referred to as GauSS-I (Gaucher Disease Severity Score Index — Type I), was recently developed for *GD type I* by DiRocco and colleagues.[36] The index includes six specific domains, representing the major sites of *GD* pathology; a

Table 4.1a. Gaucher disease scoring system.*

Skeletal Domain	Score
Bone marrow infiltration[†]	
Absent/minimal	0
Mild	1
Intermediate	2
Severe	3
Impairment of mineral component[‡]	
Absent/minimal	0
Mild	1
Intermediate	2
Severe	3
Osteonecrosis	
None	0
Medullary infarction	1
Osteonecrosis	2
Prosthesis	3
Pathologic fracture	
Absent	0
Reported	2
Hematological Domain	**Score**
Hemoglobin concentration	
>12 g/dL (male); >11.5 g/dL (female)	0
Between 10–12	1
Between 8–9.9	2
<8 or need for blood transfusion	3
WBC count	
$>4 \times 10^9/L$	0
Between 2.5–3.9	1
<2.5	2
<1.9	3

(*Continued*)

Table 4.1a. *(Continued)*

Hematological Domain	Score
Platelet count	
$>150 \times 10^9$/L	0
Between 101–150	1
Between 60–100	2
<60	3
Bleeding time	
<8 min	0
>8	1

Biomarker Domain	Score
Serum chitotriosidase	
<600 nmol/mL × h	0
600–4000	1
4001–15,000	2
>15,000	3
CCL18	
<72 ng/mL	0
72–236	1
237–1,000	2
>1,000	3

Visceral Domain	Score
Spleen	
No MRI/US lesions	0
MRI/US lesions	3
No splenectomy	0
Splenectomy	2
Volume <5 MN	0
Between 5–9	1
Between 10–15	2
>15	3
Liver	
No hepatic disease	0
Hepatic disease	3
Volume <1.25 MN	0
Between 1.25–2.5	1
Between >2.5	2

(Continued)

Table 4.1a. (*Continued*)

Pulmonary Domain	Score
Pulmonary hypertension	
Absent	0
Moderate	1
Severe	2
Respiratory failure	
Absent	0
Moderate	1
Severe	2

Neurological Domain	Score
No signs/symptoms	0
Peripheral neuropathy	1
Parkinson disease	3

*Di Rocco M, Giona F, Carubbi F, Linari S, Minichilli F, Brady RO, Mariani G, Cappellini MD. *Haematologica* 2008;93(8):1211–1218.
†Based on either MRI or scintigraphic evaluations
‡Based on either DEXA or Hermann's X-ray classification

score is assigned according to impact on morbidity, which has been shown to correlate with the Zimran SSI (an older system widely used in reports emanating primarily from European centers).[39] In contrast to the Zimran SSI, which assigns more weight (~55% of maximum total score) to complications of the disease such as splenectomy, fractures, and CNS involvement, the GauSS-I assigns only about 19% of the total score to such pathologies.[39] This is an important distinction as disease complications are irreversible and not likely to change with current treatment modalities. The sensitivity of the index to change with therapy has been assessed in 53 *GD* patients on enzyme therapy (mean duration 30 ± 17 months), and the response profile has been compared with the Zimran SSI. The mean change from baseline to follow-up observed with the GauSS-I was significantly greater (by a factor of almost 2) than the equivalent change observed using the Zimran SSI.

Given the distinct neurologic problems associated with *types II and III GD*, a separate scoring system was devised for this subgroup of patients. The proposed scoring system (Table 4.1b) was based on a

Lysosomal Storage Disorders

Table 4.1b. Neuronopathic GD severity scoring tool.*

Horizontal gaze palsy	Normal (although not likely in diagnosis)	0
	Horizontal saccades absent, vertical saccades present	1.5
	Horizontal saccades and vertical saccades absent	3
Epilepsy	No seizures	0
	Seizures not requiring anti-convulsants	1
	Seizures controlled with anti-convulsants	2
	Seizures requiring combination therapy or resistant to anti-convulsants	3
Development/cognitive ability	Normal	0
	Mildly impaired (IQ less than 85 or equivalent)	1
	Moderate (IQ between 50–57 or equivalent)	2
	Severe (more than half of their chronological age)	3
Neurology Pattern		
Ataxia/gait	Normal, apparent only on tandem walking	0
	Ataxia on straight gait, able to walk without assistance	1
	Able to walk only with assistance	2
	Unable to walk	3
Cerebellar signs/ataxia	No intention tremor	0
	Intention tremor not affecting function	1.5
	Intention tremor with marked impact on function	3
Pyramidal	Normal tone with increased reflexes	0
	Mildly to moderately increased tone and reflexes	1
	Increased tone reflexes with sustained/unsustained clonus	2
	Severe spasticity with inability to walk	3
Extra-pyramidal	Normal	0
	Variable tone and posturing not impairing function, with or without therapy	1
	Variable tone and posturing impairing function, despite therapy	2
	Significant rigidity with no/minimal benefit from therapy	3

(Continued)

Table 4.1b.   (*Continued*)

Swallowing difficulties/ oral bulbar function	Normal	0
	Mild dysphagia (excess drooling)	1
	Moderate dysphagia (risk of aspiration, modification to diet required)	2
	Severe dysphagia (requiring non-oral feeding)	3
Speech	Normal (and those too young yet to speak)	0
	Mild to moderate dysarthria impairing intelligibility to unfamiliar listener	1
	Severe dysarthria with most speech unintelligible to familiar and unfamiliar listener	2
	Anarthria	3
Ophthalmology	Normal	0
	Cranial nerve palsy (previously corrected or not)	1.5
	Cranial nerve palsy (reappearing despite surgical correction)	3
Spinal alignment (kyphosis)	Normal	0
	Mild kyphosis – but flexible	1
	Moderate kyphosis – partially corrected	2
	Severe kyphosis – fixed	3
Total		33

*Davies EH, Surtees R, DeVile C, Schoon I, Vellodi A. *J Inherit Metab Dis*. 2007;30(5):768–782.

retrospective analysis of data on 15 patients and a literature review of data on additional 102 patients.[40] The tool has several components, including the evaluation of cognitive ability, speech and swallowing problems, pyramidal and extra-pyramidal features, ophthalmologic findings and spinal alignment issues. A limitation of the tool is that it fails to incorporate the impact of systemic and visceral disease upon neurological function.

Anderson-Fabry disease (AFD). Table 4.2: The Mainz Severity Score Index (MSSI) was developed as a scoring system for measuring the severity of *AFD*, and has been used to evaluate the clinical course of the disease in patients on enzyme therapy.[41] The combination of individual components, representing the pattern of organ/system involvement, is used to

Table 4.2. Anderson-Fabry disease: the Mainz Severity Score Index (MSSI).*

General Score			Neurological Score			Cardiovascular Score			Renal Score		
Sign/symptom	Rating	Score	Sign/symptom	Rating	Score	Sign/symptom	Rating	Score	Sign/symptom	Rating	Score
Characteristic facial appearance	No	0	Tinnitus	No	0	Changes in cardiac muscle thickness	No	0	Evidence of renal dysfunction	No	0
	Yes	1		Mild	1		Thickening of wall/septum	1		Proteinuria	4
				Severe	2		LVH seen in ECG	6		Tubular dysfunction/low	8
Angiokeratoma	No	0	Vertigo	No	0		Cardiomyopathy (<15 mm)	8		GFR or creatinine clearance	12
	Some	1		Mild	1		Severe cardiomyopathy (>15 mm)	12		End-stage renal failure (serum creatinine levels >3.5 mg/dl)	18
	Extensive	2		Severe	2	Valve insufficiency	No	0		Dialysis	

(Continued)

Table 4.2. (*Continued*)

General Score			Neurological Score			Cardiovascular Score			Renal Score		
Sign/symptom	Rating	Score	Sign/symptom	Rating	Score	Sign/symptom	Rating	Score	Sign/symptom	Rating	Score
Edema	No	0	Acroparesthesia	No	0	ECG abnormalities	No	0			
	Yes	1		Occasional	3		Yes	2			
				Chronic	6	Pacemaker	No	0			
Musculoskeletal	No	0	Fever pain crisis	No	0		Yes	4			
	Yes	1		Yes	2	Hypertension	No	0			
Cornea verticillata	No	0	Cerebrovascular	No	0		Yes	1			
	Yes	1		Ischemic lesions (in MRI/CT)	1						
				TIA, migraine, etc.	3						
Diaphoresis	Normal	0		Stroke	5						
	Hypo/hyper	1									
	Anhidrosis	2									

(*Continued*)

Table 4.2. (*Continued*)

General Score			Neurological Score			Cardiovascular Score			Renal Score		
Sign/symptom	Rating	Score	Sign/symptom	Rating	Score	Sign/symptom	Rating	Score	Sign/symptom	Rating	Score
Abdominal pain	No	0	Psychiatric/ psychosocial	No	0						
	Yes	2	Depression	Yes	1						
				No	0						
			Fatigue	Yes	1						
				No	0						
Diarrhea/ constipation	No	0	Reduced activity level	No	0						
	Yes	1		Yes	1						
Hemorrhoids	No	0									
	Yes	1									
Pulmonary	No	0									
	Yes	2									
New York Heart	No	0									
Association	Class I	1									
Classification†	Class II	2									
	Class III	3									
	Class IV	4									
Maximum score	18		Maximum score	20		Maximum score	20		Maximum score	18	

*Whybra C, Kampmann C, Krummenauer F, Ries M, Mengel E, Miebach E, Baehner F, Kim K, Bajbouj M, Schwarting A, Gal A, Beck M. *Clin Genet.* 2004;65(4):299–307.

†Limitation on physical activity:

Class I — None. Ordinary physical activity does not cause undue fatigue, palpitation, dyspnea, or anginal pain but shows heart involvement in the echocardiogram.

Class II — Slight. Comfortable at rest, but ordinary physical activity results in fatigue.

Class III — Marked. Comfortable at rest, but less than ordinary physical activity causes fatigue.

Class IV — Unable to carry out any physical activity without discomfort.

calculate the total MSSI score, which is divided into three grades of severity: mild (<20), moderate (20–40), and severe (>40) disease.[41]

In a study involving 30 *AFD* patients treated with agalsidase alfa (median duration of 2.9 years), the MSSI captured the correlation between disease severity, gender and age.[42] Males as expected had a worse score than females at baseline, and showed disease progression with age. After a year of treatment, total MSSI scores were significantly lower than at baseline.[42]

Krabbe disease. Table 4.3: Escolar and co-workers devised a staging system incorporating several clinical indicators and neurophysiological and neuroimaging measures, based on a retrospective review of pre-transplant findings in 42 patients.[28] Age equivalents were used to allow

Table 4.3.   Krabbe disease.*

Stage	Description
1	Child appears to be developing normally, may show some minor inconclusive neurologic signs
2	Neurologic symptoms appear obvious to clinicians
3	Signs of moderate to severe neurologic involvement
4	Advanced disease

Group Classification	Clinical Indicator
A	Mild thumb clasp (not fixed); hypotonia of shoulder girdle; weak feeding; gastroesophageal reflux
B	Fixed thumb clasp; spasticity of extremities; predominant trunk extensor tone (any age) or trunk hypotonia (>4 mo of age), >1 of the following feeding abnormalities: difficulty latching to breast/nipple, decreased rate of nutritive suck, abnormal tongue, lip, or chin movements
C	Clinical seizures; absent of deep tendon reflexes or other abnormal reflexes; exaggerated startle; visual tracking difficulties; jerky eye movements; abnormal pupillary response
D	Severe weakness, unresponsive to stimuli, loss of primitive reflexes; sensory impairment (blindness or deafness)

*Escolar ML, Poe MD, Martin HR, Kurzberg J. *Pediatrics.* 2006;118(3): e879–e889.
Staging of disease progression is based on gross signs of neurologic disease progression as noted in patient's history.

for comparison across tests and evaluation of the acquisition of new skills. Clinical assessments focused on gross motor, cognitive, receptive and expressive language, adaptive behavior, and fine motor skills.[28] Standard neurophysiological and neuroimaging tests did not prove to be useful, whereas clinical indicators were found to best classify stage of disease.[28] Pre-transplant stage was found to be predictive of post-transplant neurodevelopmental outcome.

Sanfilippo syndrome type A (MPS-IIIA). Table 4.4: Meyer and colleagues examined the natural course of *MPS-IIIA* in a group of 71 patients and compared their observations, where possible, with the progression of the disease in 14 patients with *MPS-IIIB* and four patients with *MPS-IIIC*.[43] Assessments included a questionnaire and 4-point functional performance scoring system (FPSS), which was used to assess the degree of developmental regression over time. The FPSS domains included measurements of motor and cognitive function, and speech abilities. The total disability score (TDS) was derived from the sum of average scores for each these domains. A lower score corresponds with a greater disease severity.

Table 4.4.   Sanfilippo syndrome type A.*

Function	Performance	Score
Motor function[†]	Normal walking	3
	Clumsy walking	2
	Aided walking	1
	Wheel chair/immobile	0
Speech abilities[†]	Normal speech	3
	Impairment of speech	2
	Speech difficult to understand	1
	Loss of speech	0
Cognitive function	Normal cognitive function	3
	Deterioration of cognitive function	2
	Loss of interest in environment	1
	Unresponsiveness	0

*Meyer A, Kossow K, Gal A, Mühlhausen C, Ullrich K, Braulke T, Muschol N. *Pediatrics.* 2007; 120(5): e1255–e1261.

[†]In some patients, motor and speech development were never normal, and scoring started at a score of 2.

Late infantile neuronal ceroid lipofuscinosis (*LINCL*). Table 4.5: Worgall and co-workers at the Weill Cornell Medical Center developed a severity score for *LINCL*, based on the evaluation of neurologic, ophthalmologic, and CNS imaging (both MRI and MRS; N = 18) findings in

Table 4.5.   Late infantile neuronal ceroid lipofuscinosis: the Weill Cornell LINCL scale.*

Functional Category	Rating Criteria	Score
Feeding scale	No swallowing dysfunction	3
	Mild swallowing dysfunction	2
	Moderate swallowing dysfunction	1
	Gastrostomy-tube dependent	0
Gait scale	Normal	3
	Abnormal (spastic or bradykinetic or ataxic) but able to ambulate independently	2
	Abnormal (spastic or bradykinetic or ataxic) requiring assistance	1
	Non-ambulatory	0
Motor scale	None of myoclonus, chorea/tremor/athetosis,[†] and up-going toes	3
	One of myoclonus, chorea/tremor/athetosis,[†] and up-going toes	2
	Two of myoclonus, chorea/tremor/athetosis,[†] and up-going toes	1
	Myoclonus, chorea/tremor/athetosis,[†] and up-going toes	0
Language scale	Normal speech	3
	Abnormal speech with abnormal articulation or decreased vocabulary	2
	Barely understandable speech with severe dysarthria or very few meaningful words	1
	Unintelligible words or no speech	0
Total score	Sum of scores for feeding, gait, motor and language problems	

*Worgall S, Kekatpure MV, Heier L, Ballon D, Dyke JP, Shungu D, Mao X, Kosofsky B, Kaplitt MG, Souweidane MM, Sondhi D, Hackett NR, Hollmann C, Crystal RG. *Neurology*. 2007; 69(6):521–535.
[†]Any one of the three motor symptoms: chorea, tremor, and athetosis are considered as one scoring.

32 patients.[44] A scoring system developed by the group at Hamburg University had been in use previously, incorporating several elements such as the incidence of seizures (at 3-month intervals), motor dysfunction, language abnormality, and vision.[45] The Weill Cornell *LINCL* modification of the Hamburg scale, which focused only on the CNS manifestations, included the following additional assessments: swallowing function, gait, and motor system and speech abnormalities.[44] Thus, the Weill Cornell *LINCL* scale represents a more comprehensive neurologic assessment, and excludes events prior to the time of the assessment (such as onset of seizures). This scoring system was found to correlate better with patient age and disease duration, and with the results of brain imaging.[44] The individual assessments also separated over a wider range, and the slope of the decline with age was steeper. Thus, the system may be able to show a slower rate of decline with age more readily, and make it particularly valuable for the assessment of the effect of novel therapies.

Juvenile NCL (JNCL). A comprehensive clinical rating scale has also been developed for patients with *JNCL*, which includes assessment of motor, behavioral, and functional capability.[46] Parents were asked to complete the Child Behavior Checklist, Scales of Independent Behavior – Revised. A structured interview was also conducted to assess obsessive-compulsive symptoms. Affected children in this series were found to be limited in their ability to perform activities of daily living, including self-care, hygiene, socialization, and other age-appropriate tasks.[46] Males and females did not differ with regard to the number of behavioral and psychiatric problems.

A cross-sectional study of 15 affected children (mean age 14.3 ± 2.9 years) noted average attention performance to be significantly below age-expected normative data.[47] Longitudinal evaluation indicated significant impairment in domains of auditory attention, memory, estimated verbal intellectual function, and verbal fluency.[46] Neuropsychological impairment was significantly correlated with disease duration and motor function, and was worse among children with a positive seizure history.[46]

Niemann-Pick type C (NPC). Table 4.6a: A severity scale has been created based on evaluation of 45 patients diagnosed with *NPC*, attributed in

Table 4.6a.   NPC disability scale.*

1. Ambulation	Score	3. Language	Score
Normal	1	Normal	1
Autonomous ataxic gait	2	Mild dysarthria (understandable)	2
Outdoor assisted ambulation	3	Severe dysarthria (only comprehensible to some members of the family)	3
Indoor assisted ambulation	4	Non-verbal communication	4
Wheelchair-bound	5	Absence of communication	5
2. Manipulation	**Score**	**4. Swallowing**	**Score**
Normal	1	Normal	1
Slight dysmetria/dystonia (allows autonomous manipulation)	2	Occasional dysphagia	2
Mild dysmetria/dystonia (requires help for several tasks but is able to feed himself)	3	Daily dysphagia	3
Severe dysmetria/dystonia (requires assistance in all activities)	4	Nasogastric tube or gastric button feeding	4

*Iturriaga C, Pineda M, Fernández-Valero EM, Vanier MT, Coll MJ. *J Neurol Sci.* 2006;249(1):1–6.

30 evaluable patients with mutations in the *NPC1* gene.[48] Disease onset ranged from perinatal (N = 3) to severe infantile (7), late infantile (6), and juvenile (11), to adulthood (3). The four domains evaluated included assessments of ambulation, manipulation, language and swallowing problems. Clumsiness in children with otherwise normal motor development was found to precede the onset of ataxia by 2–4 years.[48] This disability scale could be useful for monitoring the evolution of disease, establishing possible phenotypic correlations and evaluating the effect of future therapies. A new scale (Table 4.6b) has been introduced, and assessments conducted in 37 patients showed disease to follow a linear course of progression, independent of age of onset.[49]

Table 4.6b. NPC disability scale.*

Eye Movements	Score	Ambulation	Score
Normal	0	Normal	0
Mild VSGP[†], detected by physician only	1	Clumsy	1
Functional VSGP, noted by family or compensation with head movements	2	Ataxic, unassisted gait or not walking by 18 months	2
Total VSGP, abnormal horizontal saccades may be present	3	Assisted ambulation or not walking by 24 months	4
Total ophthalmoplegia (vertical and horizontal saccades absent)	5	Wheelchair dependent	5

Speech	Score	Swallow	Score
Normal	0	Normal, no dysphagia	0
Mild dysarthria (easily understood)	1	Cough while eating	1
		Intermittent dysphagia with liquids	+1
Severe dysarthria (difficult to understand)	2	Intermittent dysphagia with solids	+1
		Dysphagia with liquids	+2
Non-verbal/functional communication skills for needs	3	Dysphagia with solids	+2
		Nasogastric or gastric tube for supplemental feeding	4
Minimal communication	5	Nasogastric or gastric tube feeding only	5

Fine Motor Skills	Score	Cognition	Score
Normal	0	Normal	0
Slightly dysmetria/dystonia (independent manipulation)	1	Mild learning delay, grade appropriate for age	1
Mild dysmetria/dystonia (requires little to no assistance, able to feed self without difficulty)	2	Moderate learning delay, individualized curriculum or modified work setting	3
Moderate dysmetria/dystonia (limited fine motor skills, difficulty feeding self)	4	Severe learning delay/plateau, no longer in school or no longer able to do work, some loss of cognitive function	4

(Continued)

Table 4.6b. (*Continued*)

Fine Motor Skills	Score	Cognition	Score
Severe dysmetria/dystonia (gross motor limitation, requires assistance for self-care activities)	5	Minimal cognitive function	5

Hearing (Sensorineural)	Score	Memory	Score
Normal (all tones ≤15 dB HL)	0	Normal	0
High frequency hearing loss (PTA ≤15 dB HL, >15 dB HL in high frequency)	1	Mild short-term or long-term memory loss	1
Slight-mild frequency hearing loss (PTA 16–44 dB HL)	2	Moderate short-term or long-term memory loss (gets lost)	2
Moderate frequency hearing loss (PTA 45–70 dB HL)	3	Difficulty following commands	3
Severe frequency hearing loss (PTA 71–90 dB HL)	4	Unable to follow commands	4
Profound frequency hearing loss (PTA >90 dB HL)	5	Minimal memory	5

Seizures	Score
None	0
History of single seizure	1
Rare seizures	2
Seizure, well controlled with meds	3
Seizure, difficult to control with meds	5

Modifiers	Score		Score
Gelastic epilepsy		Hyperreflexia	
None	0	None	0
Definitive history	+1	Mild (3+)	+1
Frequent (every months)	+2	Severe (+ clonus)	+2
Nacolepsy		Incontinence	
None	0	None	0
Definitive history	+1	Occasional	+1
Frequent (every months)	+2	Frequent	+2

(*Continued*)

Table 4.6b. (*Continued*)

Modifiers	Score		Score
Behavior		Auditory brainstem	
None	0	response (ABR)	
History of ADHD, aggressive	+1	Normal	0
Harmful to self/others	+2	Abnormal	+1
Psychiatric		Absent	+2
None	0	Respiratory	
History of mild depression	+1	None	0
History of major depression,		History of pneumonia	+1
hallucinations or	+2	Pneumonia ≥2 × /yr or active	+2
psychotic episodes		therapeutic intervention	

*Yanjanin NM, Vélez JI, Gropman A, King K, Bianconi SE, Conley SK, Brewer CC, Solomon B, Pavan MJ, Arcos-Burgos M, Patterson MC, Porter FD. *Am J Med Genet B Neuropsychiatr Genet.* 2009 May 4
†VSGP — vertical supranuclear gaze palsy

Mucopolysaccharidosis I (MPS-I). Table 4.7: A physical performance measure for affected individuals has been developed, with motor performance and endurance items. In a pilot study involving 10 patients (ages 5–29 years), increasing age was related to greater severity in physical performance and lower scores on the leg function and endurance sub-tests.[50]

Quality of Life Studies

Systematic evaluation of health-related quality of life (HRQoL), using validated instruments, has been performed in only a few cases, primarily in patients with *Gaucher disease (GD)* and *Anderson-Fabry disease (AFD)*.

In a study of 212 *GD* patients, 14 years of age and older, scores obtained on the SF-36 Health Survey were significantly worse than the age- and gender-adjusted US norms on five of the eight SF-36 sub-scales.[51] Age and joint replacement were negatively associated with physical health.[51] Patients who had been on enzyme therapy for approximately 4 years recalled four and five times more improvement in general HRQoL, when compared with recalled changes among adults in

Table 4.7a.   Physical performance measure for MPS I (MPS-PPM).*

Item	Item Description
Arm Function	
1. Simulated eating (spoon to mouth)[†]	While sitting, the subject will simulate eating by lifting a plastic spoon from table to chin 5 times.
2. Fine grasp (placing coins in a box)[†]	While sitting, the subject places 24 coins into a box (picking up one coin at a time).
3. Use of writing instrument (drawing vertical lines)[†]	While sitting, the subject uses a pencil to draw 10 straight lines on a marked paper.
4. Hand raise (weightless reach), dominant arm	While sitting, the subject lifts his/her arm up toward the ceiling.
5. Putting on a pullover shirt[†*]	While sitting, the subject puts on a pullover shirt over his/her own shirt.
6. Putting on a backpack[†]	The subject picks up a backpack from the floor (contains 10% of body weight) and puts the backpack on using proper fit position.
7. Rolling[†]	The subject rolls from back to stomach to back with arms up overhead.
Leg Function	
1. Come to sit[†]	The subject moves to a sitting position from lying on his/her back.
2. Sit to stand[†]	The subject moves from sitting in a chair to standing 5 times.
3. Pull on pants (trousers)[†]	While standing, the subject puts on a pair of pants (trousers) over his/her own pants (trousers).
4. Floor to stand[†]	The subject stands up from a cross-legged sitting position on the floor, walks 3 meters and returns to original sitting position on the floor.
5. Stand to squat and return[†]	The subject squats down, touches the floor and returns to standing 5 times.
Endurance	
1. Endurance: 3-min walk test at comfortable speed	The distance covered and the subject's maximum heart rate are recorded as the subject walks for 3 minutes at a comfortable pace.
2. Endurance: 3-min walk test at fast speed	The distance covered and the subject's maximum heart rate are recorded as the subject walks for 3 minutes at a fast pace.

*Dumas HM, Fragala MA, Haley SM, Skrinar AM, Wraith JE, Cox GF. Physical performance testing in mucopolysaccharidosis I: a pilot study. *Pediatr Rehabil.* 2004;7(2):125–131.
[†]Task must be completed in less than 1 minute.

Table 4.7b.   MPS I- Measure of physical functioning severity.*

	Score
Joint involvement	
Dominant UE Shoulder Flexion Active ROM >120°	0
Dominant UE Shoulder Flexion Active ROM limited to 91–120°	1
Dominant UE Shoulder Flexion Active ROM <90°	2
Dominant LE Active Ankle Dorsiflexion >6°	0
Dominant LE Ankle Dorsiflexion Active ROM 0–5°	1
Dominant LE Ankle Dorsiflexion Active ROM <0°	2
Ambulation	
Community ambulation without modifications (car/taxi for distances >1 mile)	0
Community ambulation with modifications (use of pushchair/stroller for distances >0.5 mile or 15 min)	1
Household ambulation (ambulation up to 50 ft/15.24 m without stopping for rest)	2
Non-ambulatory	3
Cardiorespiratory Function	
No limitations	0
Shortness of breath, increased respiratory rate with mild activity (i.e household ambulation)	1
Tracheostomy or oxygen use	2
Ventilator use	3
Total[†]	

*Dumas HM, Fragala MA, Haley SM, Skrinar AM, Wraith JE, Cox GF. Physical performance testing in mucopolysaccharidosis I: a pilot study. *Pediatr Rehabil.* 2004;7(2):125–131.
[†]MPS Severity Scale: 0 points = no limitations with scale items; 1–3 points = mild limitations; 4–6 points = moderate limitations; 7–10 points = severe limitations.

the general population and a separate cohort of patients with congestive heart failure.

In affected males with *AFD*, evaluations using the Medical Outcomes Study (MOS) SF-36 and an *AFD*-specific questionnaire revealed scores that were substantially lower across all assessed domains, when compared with that obtained for the general US population and among patients with other chronic disease states, including *GD*, end-stage renal disease, stroke and AIDS.[52] In the general population, stroke, cardiac problems and renal disease lead to substantial decrement in HRQoL.

The use of tools to assess the quality of life of affected individuals is anticipated to become increasingly valuable in ascertaining both the individual and societal costs of disease and the value derived from specific treatments, as these become available.

References

1. van der Voorn JP, Pouwels PJ, Hart AA, Serrarens J, Willemsen MA, Kremer HP, Barkhof F, van der Knaap MS. Childhood white matter disorders: quantitative MR imaging and spectroscopy. *Radiology* 2006;241(2):510–517.
2. Fellgiebel A, Keller I, Marin D, Müller MJ, Schermuly I, Yakushev I, Albrecht J, Bellhäuser H, Kinateder M, Beck M, Stoeter P. Diagnostic utility of different MRI and MR angiography measures in Fabry disease. *Neurology* 2009;72(1):63–68.
3. Palmeri S, Villanova M, Malandrini A, van Diggelen OP, Huijmans JG, Ceuterick C, Rufa A, DeFalco D, Ciacci G, Martin JJ, Guazzi G. Type I sialidosis: a clinical, biochemical and neuroradiological study. *Eur Neurol.* 2000;43(2):88–94.
4. Oner AY, Cansu A, Akpek S, Serdaroglu A. Fucosidosis: MRI and MRS findings. *Pediatr Radiol.* 2007;37(10):1050–1052.
5. Santavuori P, Vanhanen SL, Autti T. Clinical and neuroradiological diagnostic aspects of neuronal ceroid lipofuscinoses disorders. *Eur J Paediatr Neurol.* 2001;5(Suppl. A):157–161.
6. Inglese M, Nusbaum AO, Pastores GM, Gianutsos J, Kolodny EH, Gonen O. MR imaging and proton spectroscopy of neuronal injury in late-onset GM2 gangliosidosis. *AJNR Am J Neuroradiol.* 2005;26(8):2037–2042.
7. Brockmann K, Dechent P, Wilken B, Rusch O, Frahm J, Hanefeld F. Proton MRS profile of cerebral metabolic abnormalities in Krabbe disease. *Neurology.* 2003;60(5):819–825.
8. Kruse B, Hanefeld F, Christen HJ, Bruhn H, Michaelis T, Hänicke W, Frahm J. Alterations of brain metabolites in metachromatic leukodystrophy as detected by localized proton magnetic resonance spectroscopy *in vivo*. *J Neurol.* 1993;241(2):68–74.
9. Galanaud D, Tourbah A, Lehéricy S, Levegue N, Heron B, Billette de Villemeur T, Guffon N, Feillet F, Baumann N, Vanier MT, Seder F. 24 month-treatment with miglustat of three patients with Niemann-Pick disease

type C: follow up using brain spectroscopy. *Mol Genet Metab.* 2009;96(2): 55–58.

10. Varho T, Komu M, Sonninen P, Holopainen I, Nyman S, Manner T, Sillanpää M, Aula P, Lundbom N. A new metabolite contributing to N-acetyl signal in 1H MRS of the brain in Salla disease. *Neurology.* 1999;52(8):1668–1672.

11. Bonavita S, Virta A, Jeffries N, Goldin E, Tedeschi G, Schiffmann R. Diffuse neuroaxonal involvement in mucolipidosis IV as assessed by proton magnetic resonance spectroscopic imaging. *J Child Neurol.* 2003;18(7):443–449.

12. Vanhanen SL, Puranen J, Autti T, Raininko R, Liewendahl K, Nikkinen P, Santavuori P, Suominen P, Vuori L, Häkkinen AM. Neuroradiological findings (MRS, MRI, SPECT) in infantile neuronal ceroid-lipofuscinosis (infantile CLN1) at different stages of the disease. *Neuropediatrics* 2004;35:27–35.

13. Campbell PE, Harris CM, Vellodi A. Deterioration of the auditory brainstem response in children with type 3 Gaucher disease. *Neurology.* 2004;63(2): 385–387.

14. Aldosari M, Altuwaijri M, Husain AM. Brain-stem auditory and visual evoked potentials in children with Krabbe disease. *Clin Neurophysiol.* 2004; 115(7):1653–1656.

15. Inagaki M, Kaga Y, Kaga M, Nihei K. Multimodal evoked potentials in patients with pediatric leukodystrophy. *Suppl Clin Neurophysiol.* 2006;59:251–263.

16. Scaioli V, Nardocci N. A pathophysiological study of neuronal ceroid lipo-fuscinoses in 17 patients: critical review and methodological proposal. *Neurol Sci.* 2000;21(3 Suppl):S89–S92.

17. Simmons MA, Bruce IA, Penney S, Wraith E, Rothera MP. Otorhinolaryn-gological manifestations of the mucopolysaccharidoses. *Int J Pediatr Otorhinolaryngol.* 2005;69(5):589–595.

18. Palla A, Hegemann S, Widmer U, Straumann D. Vestibular and auditory deficits in Fabry disease and their response to enzyme replacement therapy. *J Neurol.* 2007;254(10):1433–1442.

19. Altarescu G, Sun M, Moore DF, Smith JA, Wiggs EA, Solomon BI, Patronas NJ, Frei KP, Gupta S, Kaneski CR, Quarrell OW, Slaugenhaupt SA, Goldin E, Schiffmann R. The neurogenetics of mucolipidosis type IV. *Neurology.* 2002;59(3):306–313.

20. Smith JA, Chan CC, Goldin E, Schiffmann R. Noninvasive diagnosis and ophthalmic features of mucolipidosis type IV. *Ophthalmology.* 2002;109(3): 588–594.

21. Collins J, Holder GE, Herbert H, Adams GG. Batten disease: features to facilitate early diagnosis. *Br J Ophthalmol.* 2006;90(9):1119–1124.

22. Harris CM, Taylor DS, Vellodi A. Ocular motor abnormalities in Gaucher disease. *Neuropediatrics.* 1999;30(6):289–293.

23. Patterson MC, Vecchio D, Prady H, Abel L, Wraith JE. Miglustat for treatment of Niemann-Pick C disease: a randomised controlled study. *Lancet Neurol.* 2007;6(9):765–772.

24. Husain AM. Neurophysiologic studies in Krabbe disease. *Suppl Clin Neurophysiol.* 2006;59:289–298.

25. Varho T, Jääskeläinen S, Tolonen U, Sonninen P, Vainionpää L, Aula P, Sillanpää M. Central and peripheral nervous system dysfunction in the clinical variation of Salla disease. *Neurology.* 2000;55(1):99–104.

26. Shapiro BE, Logigian EL, Kolodny EH, Pastores GM. Late-onset Tay-Sachs disease: the spectrum of peripheral neuropathy in 30 affected patients. *Muscle Nerve.* 2008;38(2):1012–1015.

27. Müller-Felber W, Horvath R, Gempel K, Podskarbi T, Shin Y, Pongratz D, Walter MC, Baethmann M, Schlotter-Weigel B, Lochmüller H, Schoser B. Late onset Pompe disease: clinical and neurophysiological spectrum of 38 patients including long-term follow-up in 18 patients. *Neuromuscul Disord.* 2007;17(9–10):698–706.

28. Escolar ML, Poe MD, Martin HR, Kurtzberg J. A staging system for infantile Krabbe disease to predict outcome after unrelated umbilical cord blood transplantation. *Pediatrics.* 2006; 118(3):e879–e889.

29. Davies EH, Surtees R, DeVile C, Schoon I, Vellodi A. A severity scoring tool to assess the neurological features of neuronopathic Gaucher disease. *J Inherit Metab Dis.* 2007;30(5):768–782.

30. Santamaria F, Andreucci MV, Parenti G, Polverino M, Viggiano D, Montella S, Cesaro A, Ciccarelli R, Capaldo B, Andria G. Upper airway obstructive disease in mucopolysaccharidoses: polysomnography, computed tomography and nasal endoscopy findings. *J Inherit Metab Dis.* 2007;30(5):743–749.

31. van der Ploeg AT. Monitoring of pulmonary function in Pompe disease: a muscle disease with new therapeutic perspectives. *Eur Respir J.* 2005; 26(6):984–985.

32. Pellegrini N, Laforet P, Orlikowski D, Pellegrini M, Caillaud C, Eymard B, Raphael JC, Lofaso F. Respiratory insufficiency and limb muscle weakness in adults with Pompe's disease. *Eur Respir J.* 2005;26(6):1024–1031.

33. Di Rocco M, Buzzi D, Tarò M. Glycogen storage disease type II: clinical overview. *Acta Myol*. 2007;26(1):42–44.

34. Pierre-Louis B, Kumar A, Frishman WH. Fabry disease: cardiac manifestations and therapeutic options. *Cardiol Rev*. 2009;17(1):31–35.

35. Lobo T, Morgan J, Bjorksten A, Nicholls K, Grigg L, Centra E, Becker G. Cardiovascular testing in Fabry disease: exercise capacity reduction, chronotropic incompetence and improved anaerobic threshold after enzyme replacement. *Intern Med J*. 2008;38(6):407–414.

36. Klinge L, Straub V, Neudorf U, Voit T. Enzyme replacement therapy in classical infantile Pompe disease: results of a ten-month follow-up study. *Neuropediatrics*. 2005;36(1):6–11.

37. Wokke JH, Escolar DM, Pestronk A, Jaffe KM, Carter GT, van den Berg LH, Florence JM, Mayhew J, Skrinar A, Corzo D, Laforet P. Clinical features of late-onset Pompe disease: a prospective cohort study. *Muscle Nerve*. 2008; 38(4):1236–1245.

38. Pastores GM. Musculoskeletal complications encountered in the lysosomal storage disorders. *Best Pract Res Clin Rheumatol*. 2008;22(5): 937–947.

39. Di Rocco M, Giona F, Carubbi F, Linari S, Minichilli F, Brady RO, Mariani G, Cappellini MD. A new severity score index for phenotypic classification and evaluation of responses to treatment in type I Gaucher disease. *Haematologica*. 2008;93(8):1211–1218.

40. Davies EH, Surtees R, DeVile C, Schoon I, Vellodi A. A severity scoring tool to assess the neurological features of neuronopathic Gaucher disease. *J Inherit Metab Dis*. 2007;30(5):768–782.

41. Whybra C, Kampmann C, Krummenauer F, Ries M, Mengel E, Miebach E, Baehner F, Kim K, Bajbouj M, Schwarting A, Gal A, Beck M. The Mainz Severity Score Index: a new instrument for quantifying the Anderson-Fabry disease phenotype, and the response of patients to enzyme replacement therapy. *Clin Genet*. 2004;65(4):299–307.

42. Parini R, Rigoldi M, Santus F, Furlan F, De Lorenzo P, Valsecchi G, Concolino D, Strisciuqlio P, Feriozzi S, Di Vito R, Ravaglia R, Ricci R, Morrone A. Enzyme replacement therapy with agalsidase alfa in a cohort of Italian patients with Anderson-Fabry disease: testing the effects with the Mainz Severity Score Index. *Clin Genet*. 2008;74(3):260–266.

43. Meyer A, Kossow K, Gal A, Mühlhausen C, Ullrich K, Braulke T, Muschol N. Scoring evaluation of the natural course of mucopolysaccharidosis type IIIA (Sanfilippo syndrome type A). *Pediatrics.* 2007;120(5):e1255–1261.

44. Worgall S, Kekatpure MV, Heier L, Ballon D, Dyke JP, Shungu D, Mao X, Kosofsky B, Kaplitt MG, Souweidane MM, Sondhi D, Hackett NR, Hollmann C, Crystal RG. Neurological deterioration in late infantile neuronal ceroid lipofuscinosis. *Neurology* 2007;69(6):521–535.

45. Steinfeld R, Heim P, von Gregory H, Meyer K, Ullrich K, Goebel HH, Kohlschütter A. Late infantile neuronal ceroid lipofuscinosis: quantitative description of the clinical course in patients with CLN2 mutations. *Am J Med Genet.* 2002;112:347–354.

46. Adams H, de Blieck EA, Mink JW, Marshall FJ, Kwon J, Dure L, Rothberg PG, Ramirez-Montealegre D, Pearce DA. Standardized assessment of behavior and adaptive living skills in juvenile neuronal ceroid lipofuscinosis. *Dev Med Child Neurol.* 2006;48:259–264.

47. Adams HR, Kwon J, Marshall FJ, de Blieck EA, Pearce DA, Mink JW. Neuropsychological symptoms of juvenile-onset batten disease: experiences from 2 studies. *J Child Neurol.* 2007;22(5):621–627.

48. Iturriaga C, Pineda M, Fernández-Valero EM, Vanier MT, Coll MJ. Niemann-Pick C disease in Spain: clinical spectrum and development of a disability scale. *J Neurol Sci.* 2006;249(1):1–6.

49. Yanjanin NM, Vélez JI, Gropman A, King K, Bianconi SE, Conley SK, Brewer CC, Solomon B, Pavan WJ, Arcos-Burgos M, Patterson MC, Porter FD. Linear clinical progression, independent of age of onset, in Niemann-Pick disease, type C. *Am J Med Genet B Neuropsychiatr Genet.* 2009 May 4.

50. Dumas HM, Fragala MA, Haley SM, Skrinar AM, Wraith JE, Cox GF. Physical performance testing in mucopolysaccharidosis I: a pilot study. *Pediatr Rehabil.* 2004;7(2):125–131.

51. Damiano AM, Pastores GM, Ware JE Jr. The health-related quality of life of adults with Gaucher's disease receiving enzyme replacement therapy: results from a retrospective study. *Qual Life Res.* 1998;7(5):373–386.

52. Gold KF, Pastores GM, Botteman MF, Yeh JM, Sweeney S, Aliski W, Pashos CL. Quality of life of patients with Fabry disease. *Qual Life Res.* 2002;11(4):317–327.

Vignette

MS was 6 years old when she was referred by her pediatrician to a child neurologist because of learning difficulties. At the initial visit, no focal or lateralizing motor or sensory deficits were noted, and routine evaluations were non-diagnostic. Family history at this point was not informative. By age 8, she had developed severe visual impairment, attributed to pigmentary macular degeneration. She also began to exhibit inattention and clumsiness, and had experienced several seizures. EEG revealed the presence of sharp waves and spikes. The diagnosis of *neuronal ceroid lipofuscinoses* (*NCL*) was entertained. Skin biopsy revealed the presence of lamellar membranous storage bodies in non-myelinated axons. When she was 10 years old, the molecular basis for juvenile *NCL* (*Batten disease*) was identified; subsequent genetic testing revealed MS to be a compound heterozygote for the common *Batten disease* mutation (1 kb deletion) and a private *battenin* gene defect (E17X). Tragically, her younger sister who began to demonstrate some learning disability around this time was also shown on genetic testing to be affected. Both girls receive palliative care, and 10 years on have suffered a significant decline in their overall performance.

The *NCLs* (commonly referred to as *Batten disease*) represent a group of disorders characterized by progressive visual impairment, seizures, and the loss of cognitive and motor functions. Several clinical subtypes have been delineated on the basis of age at onset. Collectively, the different *NCL* variants comprise the most common cause of inherited neurodegenerative disease in childhood, with an estimated incidence of 1 in 12,500. To date, at least seven different gene defects have been linked with *NCL*, which are disorders primarily transmitted in an autosomal recessive fashion (except for *Kufs disease*, which is an adult-onset disorder transmitted as an autosomal dominant trait). Discovery of the causal gene defects has provided insights into the putative basis of disease, although it is still not known why neuronal cells are selectively vulnerable and extra-neurologic dysfunction is not a disease feature. Two genes, namely *CLN-1* and *-2*, encode soluble lysosomal hydrolases, which justifies their inclusion with other LSDs.

Suggested Reading

Jalanko A, Braulke T. Neuronal ceroid lipofuscinoses. *Biochim Biophys Acta*. 2009;1793(4):697–709.

Pierret C, Morrison JA, Kirk MD. Treatment of lysosomal storage disorders: focus on the neuronal ceroid-lipofuscinoses. *Acta Neurobiol Exp (Wars)*. 2008;68(3):429–442.

Rakheja D, Narayan SB, Bennett MJ. The function of CLN3P, the Batten disease protein. *Genet Metab*. 2008;94(2):270.

5

Pathophysiology and Biomarkers

A decline in the efficiency of lysosomal substrate degradation or a disruption in the normal routes of intracellular substrate transport results in the accumulation of one or more by-products of cellular metabolism (Table 5.1).[1] In conjunction, there may be a reduction in the pool of metabolic precursors that are usually derived from recycled substrates, now trapped in the lysosome. A majority of LSDs are associated with and occasionally restricted to central nervous system (CNS) involvement, which is indicative of the vulnerability of neurons to lysosomal dysfunction.

The lysosome is a component of the endolysosomal system, which is closely associated with the ubiquitin-proteasomal and autophagosomal systems.[2] These interrelated units essentially comprise the cellular machinery for substrate degradation and recycling, homeostatic regulation and signal transduction. As the endocytic pathway is necessary for the maturation of autophagosomes, any disruption of this process may contribute to disease as a consequence of the metabolic gridlock often seen in LSDs. Altered trafficking of molecules through the endosomal network in these cases may lead to the sequestration of membrane rafts. Expansion of raft membranes in the endosomal system has been hypothesized to lead to inappropriate retention of cell surface receptors and consequent alterations in signaling events.[3]

In the majority of cases, deficient activity of a specific catabolic enzyme is the underlying cause of substrate storage. This could arise from mutations involving the gene which encodes either the relevant enzyme or its co-factor. Alternatively, an enzyme may not be fully functional because

Table 5.1.　Primary mechanisms of disease.

Mechanism	Disease
1. Deficient enzyme activity	
• Mutation in the encoding gene for the hydrolase	• Tay-Sachs, Gaucher, Anderson-Fabry, Niemann-Pick A
• Defective post-translational modification, leading to a functional deficiency or defect in lysosomal enzyme targeting	• Multiple sulfatide deficiency, I-cell disease (mucolipidosis II)
• Deficient co-factor (saposins), activator (GM2) or protective/ multi-subunit component (cathepsin A)	• Gaucher variant, G_{M2}-galiosidosis, AB variant, Galactosialidosis
2. Altered lysosomal environment, due to:	
• Changes in lysosomal pH, which influences the efficiency of enzyme activity or transporter function	• Mucolipidosis IV (lysosomal membrane TRP family member) • NCL3
3. Defect in late stages of endocytosis, impairment of lysosomal biogenesis, and autophagocytosis	• Niemann-Pick C1 (transmembrane protein) • Danon disease
4. Defect in carrier-mediated transport out of lysosomes	• Cystinosis, infantile sialic acid storage disease

of a defect in its post-translational modification, precluding its maturation (as seen with *multiple sulfatase deficiency** [*MSD*]), or because of failure of enzyme delivery to the lysosome (as a result of a defect in the signaling tag, *I-cell disease or ML-II*[†]).[4]

---

*In *MSD*, a mutation in the sulfatase modifying factor-1 (*SUMF-1*, which encodes the ER-localized formylglycine-generating enzyme) disrupts the activation of sulfatases, a process which requires the oxidation of a specific cysteine residue. As a consequence, there is deficient activity of several sulfatases, including arylsulfatase A and B, I2S, and steroid sulfatase.

[†]In *ML-II* (*I-cell disease*) and *ML-III* (*pseudo-Hurler polydystrophy*), defects involving subunits of GlcNac-1-phosphotransferase (in the trans-Golgi network) results in the inability to form mannose-6-phosphate, an essential recognition marker which directs the delivery of newly synthesized enzymes to the lysosome. Thus, GlcNac-1-phosphotransferase deficiency results in the mis-sorting and cellular loss of several lysosomal enzymes.

Changes in lysosomal pH, as observed in fibroblasts obtained from patients with *ML-IV* and *NCL-III* (*Batten disease*),[‡] can have an adverse influence on the lysosomal micro-environment.[4–6] As a consequence, there is impaired enzyme activity and/or a disruption of membrane transport function. Interestingly, changes in lysosomal pH have also been shown to affect the intracellular processing of amyloid β-protein, which is involved in the pathogenesis of Alzheimer's disease. Thus, these changes may have a contributory role in the neurodegenerative disease process associated with certain LSDs.

As cross-talk between various intracellular organelles is likely to exist, partly mediated by membrane fusion and fission events, changes in metabolite levels or ratios may have a detrimental effect on several aspects of endolysosomal function and cellular homeostasis. For instance, the accumulation of glycosaminoglycans (GAG) in *MPS* disorders leads to inhibition of sialidase activity.[7] Also, GAGs have been shown to interact with many proteins, including proteases, cytokines, adhesion molecules and growth factors. Thus, GAG storage may result in interference with various cellular processes.[7]

It is likely that cellular and organ dysfunction in the LSDs has a multi-factorial basis (Figure 5.1). A selection of putative disease pathways are discussed below.

Morphological Observations and Biochemical Correlates

Although intralysosomal substrate storage is usually the most apparent pathologic finding (Figure 5.2), the attendant mechanisms of disease eventually leading to tissue damage and organ dysfunction in patients with an LSD remain to be more fully elucidated.

[‡]*ML-IV* is caused by mutations in mucolipin-1 (*MCOLN1*), which encodes a protein (TRPML1) — a non-specific cation channel — involved with regulating lysosomal pH and possibly with membrane fusion/fission events. TRPML1 has been shown to associate with Hsc70 and Hsp40, which are required for chaperone-mediated autophagy, a selective pathway of protein degradation.

The *CLN3* product (CLN3P), which is defective in patients with *Batten disease*, is a highly hydrophobic protein which has not been purified; however, it has been shown to have a galactosylceramide-binding domain, which may be involved in the trafficking of CLN3P to rafts via recycling endosomes. Recent studies suggest *CLN3* mutations result in disruption of the liquid-ordered nature of lipid rafts, potentially impacting any signaling or channeling properties of palmitoylated proteins.

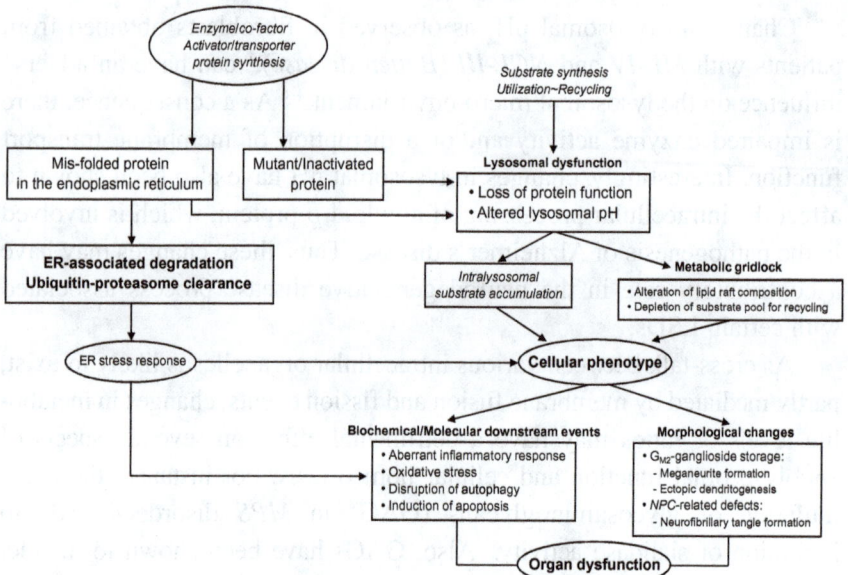

Figure 5.1. Schematic illustration of putative disease mechanisms associated with lyso-somal storage disorders.

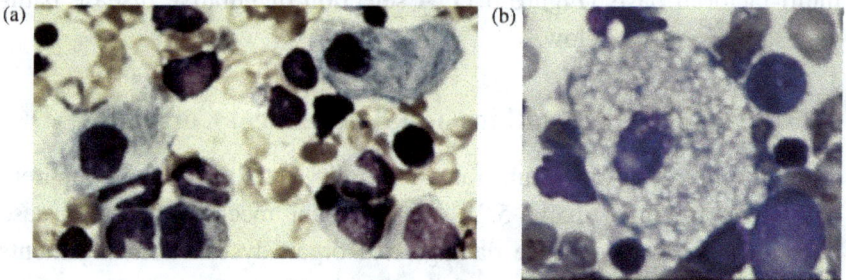

Figure 5.2. Atypical histiocytes seen in bone marrow biopsy from patients with *Gaucher disease* (a) and *Niemann-Pick disease* (b). Note: (a) 'crumpled' silk appearance; (b) foamy or soap bubble appearance.

In the pre-molecular era, the LSDs were classified according to the biochemical composition of the storage material, which led to groupings of distinct disorders into the *sphingolipidoses*, *mucopolysaccharidoses*, *glycogenoses*, *glycoproteinoses*, etc. To a large extent, clinical manifestations are correlated with sites of substrate deposition, which led to the hypothesis early on that clinical problems were mainly caused by mechanical factors and loss of cellular integrity.

In neuronal cells that have G_{M2}-ganglioside storage, there is formation of meganeurites (axonal hillock enlargements).[8] Located between the cell soma and initial portion of the axon, meganeurites may alter axonal transport and deprive distal cellular segments of trophic substances. A disruption of axonal transport may also be the basis for axonal spheroid formations (neuro-axonal dystrophy), characterized as focal enlargements of various sizes scattered along myelinated and unmyelinated axons in both the gray and white matter. Spheroids occur most commonly on GABAergic neurons, including Purkinje cells, neurons in the basal ganglia and non-pyramidal (intrinsic) cells of the cerebral cortex. In contrast to neuronal cell bodies that contain storage material, spheroids consists of collections of multi-vesicular and dense bodies, mitochondria and other organelles that would normally be transported along axons. Directed movements over long distances, as occurs in motor neurons, are microtubule dependent. Interestingly, several mutations that cause microtubule dysfunction have been implicated in motor neuron diseases.[9] Thus, defects of axonal transport may be a convergent disease pathway shared by certain LSDs with other neurogenetic entities (e.g., Charcot-Marie-Tooth disease).

Ectopic dendritogenesis (the sprouting of new synapse-covered dendritic neurites at the axon hillock) is an additional pathologic finding, limited to glycosphingolipid-storing cortical pyramidal neurons and multipolar neurons in the claustrum and amygdala.[8] Overexpression of GluR2 subunit in cultured neurons has been shown to induce ectopic dendritic spine formation, implicating AMPA receptor expression in the process of dendritic and synaptic plasticity.[10] The availability of AMPA receptors may be adversely influenced by disruptions of normal endolysosomal function. Additionally, disturbance of growth factor signaling may also be involved, based on the observation that addition of BDNF to young cortical neurons can cause the exuberant growth of dendrites.[11] These changes may have an effect on the functional maturation of neurons, or the maintenance of neuronal viability.

Primary ganglioside accumulation, mainly of G_{M2}- and G_{M3}-gangliosides, is found in the *gangliosidoses* (*Tay-Sachs* and *Sandhoff disease*). Ganglioside deposits have also been found in the *mucopolysaccharidoses (MPS)*, α*-mannosidosis* and *Niemann-Pick type C (NPC)*.[12] In the *MPS* disorders, the storage of GAGs can lead to inhibition of the activity of several ganglioside-degrading lysosomal enzymes; although it is interesting to note that the sequestered gangliosides do not typically localize with GAG storage. In any case, the resultant accumulation of gangliosides in the *MPS* is believed to contribute to the neurodegenerative process. Additionally, increased intracellular β-amyloid peptide is seen in the brain of patients with *MPS-I* and *III*, in the absence of neurofibrillary tangles (NFT) or tau-positive lesions.[13] Conversely, heparan sulphate (HS) and HS proteogylcans, which accumulate in several *MPS* disorders, have been demonstrated in Alzheimer disease (AD) plaques and other CNS lesions in amyloid-related and prion diseases.[14] These observations suggest a multi-factorial basis for the neurologic problems that afflict *MPS* patients, which may involve pathogenic mechanisms shared with other neurodegenerative diseases such as AD.

In addition to the lysosomal storage of GAGs and glycosphingolipid, there is accumulation of subunit C of mitochondrial ATP synthase (SCMAS) in the *MPS-IIIB* mouse brain.[15] Accumulation of SCMAS is also seen in various forms of *neuronal ceroid lipofuscinosis (NCL)*, in cases resulting from mutations in *CLN2–9*.[16] In contrast, sphingolipid activator protein (SAP) build-up are found in those with mutations of *CLN1* and *CTSD (cathepsin D deficiency)*.[16] The basis for this difference in the nature of the stored protein in the various *NCL* subtypes is unknown. SAP deficiency disrupts the lysosomal hydrolysis of several substrates, and it is uncertain whether this may be a factor in the neurodegeneration seen in the *NCLs*.

In *NPC*, the ganglioside build-up is believed to result from a disruption in the retro-endocytic movement of this substrate, which leads to cholesterol sequestration.[12] Interestingly, NFTs (consisting of phosphorylated microtubular proteins) have been found in *NPC* brains.[17] Indeed, immunocytochemical and Western blot analysis reveal findings in *NPC* that are indistinguishable from those found in AD. These observations suggest similar factors may be involved in the formation of NFTs seen in both *NPC* and the early stages of AD. Cathepsin D, which cleaves microtubule-associated protein tau, is increased in the brain of the *NPC* mouse model and may be a contributory factor. Studies in the chimeric *NPC* mouse, which has both wild-type and mutant Purkinje cells, indicate loss primarily of the mutant cells and retention of wild-type cells (that are unable to rescue mutant cells); suggesting there are cell-specific factors responsible for the selective vulnerability of the mutant cells. At present, the identity of these factors is unknown. Studies indicate cerebellar Purkinje neurons, a major site of neurosteroidogenesis express higher levels of the NPC1 protein than neurons from other brain regions.

Pathologic brain studies in patients with *Krabbe disease* reveal a rapid disappearance of myelin and myelin-forming cells, with reactive astrocytic gliosis and tissue infiltration by multinucleated macrophages ("globoid cells").[18] In patients with *MLD* and peripheral neuropathy, nerve biopsy reveals the typical prismatic and tuffstone inclusions in Schwann cells.[19] In *Anderson-Fabry disease*, lipid deposits are evident in ganglion cells of the dorsal root and autonomic nervous system, and in specific cortical and brainstem structures.[19] It is possible that the tissue deposits are intrinsically inert, and although they may be a sign of disease, they are essentially not an important factor in the evolving disease process.

There is great interest in defining the putative downstream events that may ultimately be responsible for disease expression, and also explain the overlap in clinical features seen in several LSDs. Several observations indicate aberrant inflammatory responses may be a disease mechanism that is common to several LSDs. Oxidative stress and other secondary pathomechanisms that have been implicated in the LSDs are listed in Table 5.2.

Biochemical and Molecular Observations

The primary and secondary substrates that accumulate in tissues of patients with an LSD have been well characterized; however, knowledge regarding the subsequent steps in pathogenesis remains incomplete.

Table 5.2. Putative mechanisms of disease.

1. Altered trafficking of molecules through the endolysosomal network, including sequestration of membrane rafts, leading to a disruption in signaling
2. Aberrant inflammatory response, either through activation of resident microglia and/or recruitment of and activation of peripheral monocytes
3. Oxidative stress and activation of ER-stress response
4. Disruption of autophagy
5. Initiation of apoptosis

In *cystinosis* and *sialic acid storage disorders*, there is a defect in carrier-mediated transport of metabolites out of the lysosome, as a result of mutations in the respective transmembrane proteins, cystinosin and sialin.[20] Other defects involving a lysosomal membrane protein include a putative cobalamin transporter (*cobalamin F type disease*) and a hybrid transporter/transferase of acetyl groups, HGSNAT (*MPS-IIIC*), and possibly the CLN7 protein (dysfunctional in the *late-infantile type of NCL*) and mucolipin (*ML-IV*).[20] Lysosomal membrane proteins are engaged in several cellular events, such as lumen acidification, metabolite export, molecular motor recruitment and organelle fusion. Molecular defects thereof, can thus lead to alterations of cellular homeostasis.

In *Anderson-Fabry disease*, increased Gb3 and other glycosphin-golipids, which accumulate as a consequence of α-galactosidase A deficiency, have been found in the caveolar fraction of endothelial cells of the mouse model.[21] This suggests that altered lipid rafts in caveolae may be involved in the altered vascular reactivity and other changes seen in this condition.

The basis for the selective vulnerability of certain cell types is not fully understood. In *GD*, glucosylceramide storage in cells of monocytic lineage is associated with chronic macrophage activation. Altered lipid composition in detergent-resistant membranes has been demonstrated in a cellular model, leading to the transformation of the lipid-engorged cells into alternatively activated macrophages with altered immuno-reactive behavior.[22,23] These changes may be relevant in relation to the increased risk for multiple myeloma seen in *GD* patients.

Observations relating to other pathogenic phenomenon described in various LSDs are briefly summarized:

1. *Neurotoxicity and aberrant inflammation*

Galactosylceramide and sulfatides, substrates that accumulate in *Krabbe disease* and *metachromatic leukodystrophy* (*MLD*), respectively, are components of the myelin membrane. Loss of myelin integrity forms the basis for the demyelination of the central and peripheral nervous system encountered in these conditions. Additionally, in *Krabbe disease* there is accumulation of galactosylsphingosine (psychosine), a lysolipid believed to promote energy depletion, the loss of oligodendrocytes, and induction of gliosis and aberrant inflammation by astrocytes in the CNS.[24] Recently, psychosine has also been shown to down-regulate AMP-activated protein kinase (AMPK), the "cellular energy switch" in oligodendrocytes and astrocytes.[25] In an oligodendrocyte cell line (MO3.13) and primary astrocytes, psychosine accumulation increased the biosynthesis of lipids, including cholesterol and free fatty acid. These findings delineate an explicit role for AMPK in psychosine-induced inflammation in astrocytes, without directly affecting the cell death of oligodendrocytes.[25] Interestingly, astrocyte dysfunction has also been demonstrated in several leukodystrophies, such as Alexander disease and megalencephalic leukoencephalopathy with subcortical cysts (MLC),[26] disorders that are not associated with lysosomal substrate storage. Again, further studies may reveal convergent disease processes in different disorders associated with neurodegeneration.

Moreover, exposure of the MO3.13 cell line to exogenous psychosine has been associated with up-regulation of JNK AP-1 (a pro-apoptotic pathway mediator) and down-regulation of the NF-κB pathway (an anti-apoptotic pathway factor).[27] In studies of a mouse-derived oligodendrocyte progenitor cell line (OLP-II), psychosine was shown to be cytotoxic in a dose-dependent manner, with resultant activation/cleavage of initiator caspase-8 and -9, and effector caspase-3. T-lymphocytes immunoreactive for LCA, UCHL-1 and CD3 were found increased around the vessels in the white matter of affected patients,[27] which suggest that immunoreactive changes may partly be involved in the myelin breakdown and glial pathology in *Krabbe disease*.

In the other LSDs, several findings also support a putative role for inflammation:

- G_{MI}-*gangliosidosis*: Studies in the mouse model have shown that G_{MI}-ganglioside accumulation induces several cellular changes, including the activation of the unfolded protein response (UPR), up-regulation of BiP and CHOP and activation of JNK2 and caspase-12.[28] These factors are likely to be involved in promoting neuronal apoptosis and aberrant inflammatory responses.
- *Sandhoff disease* (*SD*): Activated microglia has been found in the brain of the *SD* mouse model, noted to precede the massive apoptosis which

develops.[29] Involvement of microglia has also been suggested in mouse models of *MLD* and *NPC*. In the *NPC* model, studies have also shown activation of astrocytes; although the astroglial reaction has been found to coincide with up-regulation of the cytokine interleukin-1. The latter finding suggests that astrocyte activation in this case may be more likely a consequence rather than cause of the neuronal degeneration.[30]

- *Gaucher disease*: In the fetal mice brains, elevated levels of the pro-inflammatory cytokines IL-1α, IL-1β, IL-6, and TNF-α have been detected.[31] Levels of secreted nitric oxide and reactive oxygen species in the brains of the affected mouse were also higher than in wild-type mouse.[31]

- *MPS*: Examination of brains of the *MPS-I* (α-L-iduronidase deficiency) and *IIIB* (α-N-acetylglucosaminidase deficiency) mouse models revealed a subset of microglia with large storage vacuoles.[32] In addition, a profusion of cells carrying the macrophage CD68/macrosialin antigen were found in the cortex. Moreover, there was elevation in the levels of ten other transcripts associated with macrophage functions, including complement C4, three subunits of complement C1q, lysozyme M, cathepsins S and Z, cytochrome b558 small subunit, macrophage-specific protein 1, and DAP12.[32] An increase in IFN-α receptor was also observed by immunohistochemistry.[32] Taken together, these observations are suggestive of either activation of resident microglia or an influx and activation of peripheral monocytes, or both. However, it is not certain whether these changes are the consequence primarily of ganglioside storage seen in these conditions, or from GAG accumulation, or both.

Mediators of inflammation may also be involved in the pathophysiology of the bone and joint disease in *MPS*. Findings in *MPS-VI* show changes similar to those observed in osteoarthritis and rheumatoid arthritis. For instance, articular chondrocytes in the mouse model were found to undergo a high rate of apoptosis, likely to be caused by increased TGF-β, ultimately leading to marked depletion of joint proteoglycan and collagen.[33] *MPS* chondrocytes have also been shown to produce increased amounts of the cytokines interleukin-1β and tumor necrosis factor-α as well as nitric oxide, with a concomitant up-regulation of matrix metalloproteinases-2 and -9, and up-regulation of TIMP-1 (tissue inhibitor of metalloproteinase).[33] These changes may promote cartilage degeneration, and partly explain the skeletal dysplasia encountered in these conditions.

- *NCL*: Analysis of gene expression profiles of whole brain obtained from the *PPT1*-knockout (*NCL1*) mouse at various ages (from 3 to 8 months), revealed several immediate early genes (*Arc, Cyr61, c-fos, jun-b, btg2, NR4A1*) were up-regulated during the pre-symptomatic period.[34] Subsequently, immune response genes dominated, and chemokine ligands and protease inhibitors were among the most transcriptionally-responsive genes.[34] Neuronal survival factors (IGF-1 and CNTF) and a negative regulator of neuronal apoptosis (DAP kinase-1) were found to be up-regulated in the late course of the disease. There were a few genes that were down-regulated, including the $\alpha2$ subunit of the GABA-A receptor (a component of cortical and hippocampal neurons) and Hes5 (a transcription factor important in neuronal differentiation).[34]

Further investigations are required to clarify the significance of these findings in humans, but the observed changes delineate the putative sequence of events that may underlie the neurodegenerative and other disease process characteristic of these LSDs.

2. Activation of ER-stress response, oxidative stress and apoptosis

Failure to metabolize gangliosides creates a metabolic trafficking problem, and substrate build-up in the endoplasmic reticulum (ER), which normally contains little or no gangliosides. As a consequence, there is depletion of calcium stores and activation of the ER-stress response, as shown in G_{M1}-gangliosidosis.[35] In G_{M2}-gangliosidosis, increased gangliosides in microsomal membranes have been shown to inhibit SERCA, leading to ER stress.[36] In *GD*, enhanced calcium release from the ER in response to glutamate has been described.[37] These changes are believed to ultimately provoke apoptosis. Changes in calcium concentration across neuronal membranes potentially lead to excitotoxicity, as an added mechanism of disease.

Accumulation of Gb3 in *Anderson-Fabry disease* vascular endothelium is associated with increased production of reactive oxygen species (ROS) and increased expression of cell adhesion molecules.[38] *In vitro* studies also show that Gb3-loading results in increased intracellular ROS production in cultured vascular endothelial cells in a dose-dependent manner, and lead to induction of the expression of intercellular adhesion molecule-1, vascular cell adhesion molecule-1, and E-selectin.[38] These observations may partly explain the altered vascular reactivity described in *AFD* patients.

In studies involving fibroblasts obtained from patients with various LSDs, extraordinary sensitivity to brefeldin-A-induced apoptosis has been observed, which suggests pre-existing ER stress conditions.[39] These pathogenetic events may be a potential target that is amenable to treatment by pharmacologic chaperones (see Chapter 6).

3. *Autophagy and associated defects*

Autophagy is a lysosomal-dependent catabolic process through which long-lived cytosolic proteins and organelles (such as mitochondria) are sequestered by double-membrane vesicles and ultimately degraded after fusion with lysosomes.[40] Autophagy is also microtubule-dependent; thus, disruption of microtubule function leading to a defect in autophagy may be a pathologic event implicated in the LSDs. Abnormal autophagy results in the cellular accumulation of toxic substrates (including ubiquitinated proteins, p62) that mediate cell death. Recently, increased levels and aggregation of p62 were observed in *ML-IV* fibroblasts, suggesting that abnormal accumulation of ubiquitinated protein inclusions may contribute to the phenotype observed in this condition.[41]

Studies in the mouse models of *MSD* and *MPS-IIIA* also suggest defects in autophagy. In affected cells, reduced co-localization of the lysosomal membrane protein LAMP-1 with the autophagosome marker LC3 indicates an impairment of lysosome/autophagosome fusion.[42] These observations were coupled with a decreased ability to degrade aggregate-prone proteins, and the accumulation of polyubiquitinated proteins and non-functional mitochondria. In *NPC*, there is increased expression of Beclin-1 and LC3-II, and Purkinje neuron cell death in this disorder is believed to be dependent on autophagy.[44] The alterations in autophagy in *NPC* were associated with GSK3β, suggesting an mTOR-independent induction of autophagy. Accumulation of autophagic vacuoles in the heart and skeletal muscle are hallmarks of *Danon disease*.[44] LAMP2, which is defective in *Danon disease*, is believed to be involved in lysosome/ autophagosome fusion, and may have a role in dynein-based centripetal motility. A disturbance of autophagy has also been found in the mouse model of *Pompe disease*,[45] which interestingly has been linked to a deficiency in the trafficking/processing of recombinant enzyme along the endocytic pathway.

The other main pathway responsible for the efficient degradation and turnover of proteins within the cell is the ubiquitin-proteasome system (UPS).[46] Aggregate formation inhibits proteasomal degradation of proteins, a factor implicated in disorders associated with polyglutamine repeats, such as the spinocerebellar ataxias. Mutant proteins that are mis-folded in the ER are detected by a protein quality control system, undergo ER-associated degradation and ultimately are directed to the UPS. As a consequence, there may be ER and oxidative stress, and a concomitant loss of enzyme activity within the lysosome.

Miscellaneous Findings

In the *MPS* disorders, there is a disturbance of sequential glycosamino-glycans (GAG) degradation; GAGs are heteropolysaccharides that contain repeating disaccharide units, which are components of cartilage and bone. Defects in GAG metabolism and the resultant changes in cellular homeostasis lead to a disturbance of skeletal development (dysos-tosis), and degenerative joint disease and contractures.[7]

Abnormalities in collagen organization in various tissues obtained from *MPS* patients have been described. In a patient with *Scheie syndrome (MPS-IS)*, investigations of collagen architecture by transmission electron microscopy and synchroton X-ray diffraction revealed sulfated GAG deposits in the cornea that disrupted the extracellular matrix.[47] Similar find-ings have been described in animal models of *MPS,* and these changes may be the basis for corneal opacities, which is a common feature of *MPS*.[48]

Impairment of elastic fiber assembly has also been observed in fibrob-lasts from patients with *MPS-I*, but not in *MPS-III*.[49] It has been hypothesized that these findings may be due to functional inactivation of a key protein (elastin binding protein, EBP), as a result of the build-up of dermatan sulfate-containing moieties.[49] Interestingly, these changes can be reversed in tissue culture by overexpression of versican, a chondroitin sulfate proteoglycan. Studies in the *MPS-I* mouse suggest up-regulation of elastin-degrading proteins (MMP-12 and cathepsin S), which are mediated by STATs. The resultant elastin fragmentation may be the basis for aortic dilatation and valve disease.[50]

Impaired elastogenesis has also been described in other LSDs resulting from a deficiency of β-galactosidase (β-Gal), protective protein/cathepsin A (PPCA) or neuraminidase-1 (NEU1 or sialidase) activity.[51,52] In β-Gal deficiency disorders (G_{MI}-*gangliosidosis* and *Morquio syndrome, MPS-IVB*), mutations within the encoding gene for β-Gal affect EBP transcription, as the gene for EBP is embedded within the same locus. EBP acts as a chaperone for tropoelastin, and is a component of the receptor complex which includes PPCA and NEU1; this multi-subunit complex is impaired in *galactosialidosis*.[52] It has been postulated that NEU1 normally catalyzes the removal of terminal sialic acids from microfibrillar glycoproteins and other adjacent matrix glycoconjugates, unmasking their penultimate galactosugars. In turn, these exposed galactosugars interact with the galectin domain of EBP, inducing the release of transported tropoelastin molecules and facilitating their subsequent assembly into elastic fibers. These observations may explain the skeletal and connective tissue problems noted in these LSD subtypes, which overlap with the bone and joint architectural changes encountered in the *MPS*.

In *ML-IV*, there may be aberrant sorting and/or traffic along the late endosome-lysosome pathway, as a consequence of mutations in the *MCOLN1* gene.[53] Alternatively, it has been suggested that the gene product mucolipin-1, an integral membrane protein which may function as a Ca^{2+} permeable channel, or an outwardly rectifying monovalent cation channel regulated by either Ca^{2+} or lysosomal pH, may be involved with regulating lysosomal acidification.[54] In this case, defect of *MCOLN1* can be envisaged as leading to a failure of generalized hydrolysis, which may explain the varied lysosomal accumulations, consisting of phospholipids, sphingolipids and GAGs that are seen in the tissues of affected individuals.

In *NPC*, studies of brain from affected mice revealed deficient allopregnanolone, a neurosteroid which requires cholesterol for its synthesis.[55] This observation suggests lysosomal sequestration of cholesterol limits its availability in the mitochondria, wherein the synthetic enzymes for allopreganolone are found. As neurosteroids are known modulators of neurogenesis and neuronal survival, deficient concentrations of these substances are likely to be detrimental. Recently, allopregnanolone treatment of fibroblasts from *NPC* patients or *NPC1* deficient cells has been observed to reduce levels of ROS species and lipid peroxidation, and prevent peroxide-induced apoptosis and NF-κB activation.[56] Thus, allopregnanolone supplementation may be one therapeutic approach to consider for *NPC*.

Biomarkers and Their Roles in Assignment of Disease Activity or Severity, and Changes in Patient Profile in Response to Therapy

There is an active interest in identifying biomarkers that can serve as a surrogate for or indicator of disease severity, in terms of either overall disease burden or involvement of a particular organ/system. Ideally, a biomarker should be easily and cheaply measurable in samples, such as blood or urine, which can be readily obtained. Also, the biomarker concentration or activity should be found to be greatly elevated in diseased states, without overlap in values between affected and healthy subjects, and should change rapidly in response to specific treatment outcomes that are clinically meaningful.

Mucopolysaccharidosis: Deficient α-L-iduronidase (IDUA) activity, the cause of *MPS-I*, results in the accumulation of dermatan and heparan sulphate. The levels of oligosaccharides derived from GAGs in cultured *MSP-I* fibroblasts (as measured by electrospray ionization tandem mass spectrometry), when combined with residual IDUA activity, has been shown to distinguish *MPS-I* patients with and without CNS involvement.[57] The practical application of these techniques in the final assignment of disease subtype remains to be determined, but may be useful when combined with genotype information in the selection of appropriate therapy (stem cell transplantation versus enzyme therapy) for patients with *MPS* (see Chapter 6).

Recently, serum heparin co-factor II-thrombin complex (HCII-TC) has been found to be elevated in untreated MPS patients, and serum

HCII-TC levels appeared to correlate with disease severity.[58] HCII-TC is a GAG regulated serpin–protease complex. In the *MPS* disorder where specific enzyme therapy is available (i.e., *Types I, II, and VI*), serum levels of HCII-TC declined in response to treatment, but not to levels found in controls.

Analysis by SELDI-TOF mass spectrometry of plasma from *MPS* patients has revealed an increase in the ratio of ApoCI':ApoCI, attributed to an increase in the activity of dipeptidyl peptidase IV (DPP-IV).[59] DPP-IV activity decreased during the first 10 weeks of ERT in *MPS-I* patients. DPP-IV has an important regulatory role in metabolism, including modulation of the activity of neuropeptides, hormones, cytokines and chemokines. It is possible that DPP-IV elevation could cause some of the secondary pathology in *MPS*, and inhibition of DPP-IV might have a role in *MPS* therapy.

Gaucher disease: In untreated patients, plasma glucosylceramide (GlcCer) levels are increased (on average ~3-fold), and changes in GlcCer/Cer ratio have been correlated with disease severity.[60] Enzyme therapy and substrate reduction therapy (SRT) resulted in decreased plasma GlcCer levels as early as 6 months of treatment; incidentally, the observed changes were noted to be most robust in treated patients with a pronounced clinical response.

In addition, several markers, including chitotriosidase, CCL18/PARC and MIP-α and -β, have been found to be elevated in serum of patients with *GD*.[61] Plasma chitotriosidase activity was also correlated with abnormal bone marrow infiltration, which is modified by enzyme therapy, in a pattern indicative of a dose-response relationship. Unfortunately, up to 6% of the European and North American population are null for chitotriosidase activity, and about 30% are heterozygous for an inactivating intragenic duplication in the chitotriosidase gene; thus, CCL18/PARC may be a more informative marker to follow in *GD* patients. CCL18/PARC concentrations have been correlated with visceral volumes, and shown to decline with therapy. A correlation has also been established between the osteoclast-activating cytokines (MIP1-α and -β) and skeletal involvement in *GD*. Other markers known to be elevated in GD include angiotensin-converting enzyme (ACE), tartrate-resistant acid phosphate (TRAP) and ferritin.

Several markers of bone turnover are also altered in patients with *GD*, although their clinical utility has not been established. In one study, plasma interleukin-18 concentration has been correlated with two bone formation markers (bone-specific alkaline phosphatase activity and osteocalcin concentration), and macrophage colony-stimulating factor (M-CSF) concentration with the bone absorption marker of *N*-telopeptide to helix in urine.[62]

Anderson-Fabry disease: Elevated levels of a deacylated globotriaosylceramide (lysoGb3) have been found in the plasma of classically affected *AFD* males and in tissues of *AFD* mice.[63] LysoGb3 has been shown to inhibit AGAL activity, and exposure of smooth muscle cells to lysoGb3 promotes tissue proliferation, which may be the basis for the increased intima-media thickness seen in *AFD* patients. The presence of lysoGb3 in the plasma of females who carry the *AFD* mutation, which has been found to correlate with left ventricular hypertrophy, may explain the development of symptoms among heterozygotes,[63] but this observation requires further investigation.

Prior studies had shown plasma and urine Gb3 levels to be elevated in *AFD* patients, and declined with enzyme therapy.[64,65] However, no correlation has been established between Gb3 concentration in plasma or tissue and disease severity. Indeed, the amount of Gb3 storage in cardiomyopathic hearts from *AFD* patients only comprises <2% of its weight. Therefore, other mechanism may be involved. Abnormal cardiac extracellular matrix turnover may be a factor which contributes to the development of cardiac disease in *AFD*. Affected individuals have been shown to have high serum levels of matrix metalloproteinase-9, which was correlated with systolic function (based on endocardial and mid-wall fractional shortening) that was shown to be independent of age and sex.[66]

Recently, abnormal expression and processing of uromodulin has been described in *AFD*, and shown to reflect tubular cell storage alterations.[67] Immunohistochemical analysis revealed abnormal uromodulin localization in the thick ascending limb of Henle's loop and the distal convoluted tubule.[67] These changes were associated with decreased urinary uromodulin excretion, which was found to be reversed by enzyme therapy and SRT. Additional studies are required to confirm these observations, that may partly be relevant to changes that promote the development of renal disease in *AFD* patients.

Pompe disease: Urinary Glc4 and plasma Hex4 levels have been shown to be increased in patients with *Pompe disease*.[68] Levels of these markers decreased after initiation of enzyme therapy, and patients with the best overall response showed a decrease in marker levels to within, or near, normal values.[68]

As validated measures of disease severity become available and correlation studies are performed, the role of biomarkers as surrogate indicators of disease burden and their role in monitoring therapeutic response will be clarified. Meanwhile, on-going efforts, employing various strategies such as SELDI-TOF-MS as a proteomic-based screening tool, are anticipated to reveal markers that will help with prediction of disease severity and that may also be useful in monitoring of therapy.[69] Protein profiling provides an opportunity to identify and analyze multiple markers, and enables a systems biology approach to ascertain the impact of the primary deficiency in lysosomal function. However, the amount of information that can be generated is enormous, and presents a major challenge with interpretation and determination of the clinical significance of the findings. Furthermore, it is likely that any protein whose concentration or activity may be modified during a disease state is influenced by disease stage, and by therapeutic interventions put into place. These and other concerns necessitate the need to validate initial observations, prior to implementation in general practice.

References

1. Ballabio A, Gieselmann V. Lysosomal disorders: from storage to cellular damage. *Biochim Biophys Acta*. 2009;1793(4):684–696.
2. Todde V, Veenhuis M, van der Klei IJ. Autophagy: principles and significance in health and disease. *Biochim Biophys Acta*. 2009;1792(1):3–13.
3. Simons K, Gruenberg J. Jamming the endosomal system: lipid rafts and lysosomal storage diseases. *Trends Cell Biol*. 2000;10(11):459–456.
4. Dierks T, Schlotawa L, Frese MA, Radhakrishnan K, von Figura K, Schmidt B. Molecular basis of multiple sulfatase deficiency, mucolipidosis

II/III and Niemann-Pick C1 disease — lysosomal storage disorders caused by defects of non-lysosomal proteins. *Biochim Biophys Acta.* 2009; 1793(4):710–725.

5. Venugopal B, Mesires NT, Kennedy JC, Curcio-Morelli C, Laplante JM, Dice JF, Slaugenhaupt SA. Chaperone-mediated autophagy is defective in mucolipidosis type IV. *J Cell Physiol.* 2009;219(2):344–353.

6. Holopainen JM, Saarikoski J, Kinnunen PK, Järvelä I. Elevated lysosomal pH in neuronal ceroid lipofuscinoses (NCLs). *Eur J Biochem.* 2001;268(22): 5851–5856.

7. Clarke LA. The mucopolysaccharidoses: a success of molecular medicine. *Expert Rev Mol Med.* 2008 Jan 18;10:e1.

8. Walkley SU. Pathogenic cascades in lysosomal disease — Why so complex? *J Inherit Metab Dis.* 2009;32(2):181–189.

9. El-Kadi AM, Soura V, Hafezparast M. Defective axonal transport in motor neuron disease. *J Neurosci Res.* 2007;85(12):2557–2566.

10. Passafaro M, Nakagawa T, Sala C, Sheng M. Induction of dendritic spines by an extracellular domain of AMPA receptor subunit GluR2. *Nature.* 2003;424: 677–681.

11. McAllister KA. Cellular and molecular mechanisms of dendrite growth. *Cerebral Cortex.* 2001;10:963–973.

12. Walkley SU, Vanier MT. Secondary lipid accumulation in lysosomal disease. *Biochim Biophys Acta.* 2009;1793(4):726–736.

13. Ginsberg SD, Galvin JE, Lee VM, Rorke LB, Dickson DW, Wolfe JH, Jones MZ, Trojanowski JQ. Accumulation of intracellular amyloid-beta peptide (A beta 1–40) in mucopolysaccharidosis brains. *J Neuropathol Exp Neurol.* 1999;58(8):815–824.

14. Su JH, Cummings BJ, Cotman CW. Localization of heparan sulfate glycosaminoglycan and proteoglycan core protein in aged brain and Alzheimer's disease. *Neuroscience.* 1992;51(4):801–813.

15. Ryazantsev S, Yu WH, Zhao HZ, Neufeld EF, Ohmi K. Lysosomal accumulation of SCMAS (subunit c of mitochondrial ATP synthase) in neurons of the mouse model of mucopolysaccharidosis III B. *Mol Genet Metab.* 2007;90(4):393–401.

16. Jalanko A, Braulke T. Neuronal ceroid lipofuscinoses. *Biochim Biophys Acta.* 2009;1793(4):697–709.

17. Suzuki K, Parker CC, Pentchev PG, Katz D, Ghetti B, D'Agostino AN, Carstea ED. Neurofibrillary tangles in Niemann-Pick disease type C. *Acta Neuropathol.* 1995;89(3):227–238.

18. Hörster F, Surtees R, Hoffmann GF. Disorders of intermediary metabolism: toxic leukoencephalopathies. *J Inherit Metab Dis.* 2005;28(3):345–356.

19. Takahashi K, Naito M. Lipid storage disease: Part II. Ultrastructural pathology of lipid storage cells in sphingolipidoses. *Acta Pathol Jpn.* 1985; 35(2): 385–408.

20. Ruivo R, Anne C, Sagné C, Gasnier B. Molecular and cellular basis of lysosomal transmembrane protein dysfunction. *Biochim Biophys Acta.* 2009; 1793(4):636–649.

21. Shu L, Shayman JA. Caveolin-associated accumulation of globotriaosylceramide in the vascular endothelium of alpha-galactosidase A null mice. *J Biol Chem.* 2007;282:20960–20967.

22. Hein LK, Duplock S, Hopwood JJ, Fuller M. Lipid composition of microdomains is altered in a cell model of Gaucher disease. *J Lipid Res.* 2008;49(8):1725–1734.

23. Boven LA, van Meurs M, Boot RG, Mehta A, Boon L, Aerts JM, Laman JD. Gaucher cells demonstrate a distinct macrophage phenotype and resemble alternatively activated macrophages. *Am J Clin Pathol.* 2004;122(3):359–369.

24. Giri S, Khan M, Rattan R, Singh I, Singh AK. Krabbe disease: psychosine-mediated activation of phospholipase A2 in oligodendrocyte cell death. *J Lipid Res.* 2006;47(7):1478–1492.

25. Giri S, Khan M, Nath N, Singh I, Singh AK. The role of AMPK in psychosine mediated effects on oligodendrocytes and astrocytes: implication for Krabbe disease. *J Neurochem.* 2008;105(5):1820–1833.

26. Gorospe JR, Maletkovic J. Alexander disease and megalencephalic leukoencephalopathy with subcortical cysts: leukodystrophies arising from astrocyte dysfunction. *Ment Retard Dev Disabil Res Rev.* 2006;12(2):113–122.

27. Zaka M, Rafi MA, Rao HZ, Luzi P, Wenger DA. Insulin-like growth factor-1 provides protection against psychosine-induced apoptosis in cultured mouse oligodendrocyte progenitor cells using primarily the PI3K/Akt pathway. *Mol Cell Neurosci.* 2005;30(3):398–407.

28. Tessitore A, del P Martin M, Sano R, Ma Y, Mann L, Ingrassia A, Laywell ED, Steindler DA, Hendershot LM, d'Azzo A. GM1-ganglioside-mediated activation of the unfolded protein response causes neuronal death in a neurodegenerative gangliosidosis. *Mol Cell.* 2004;15(5):753–766.

29. Wada R, Tifft CJ, Proia RL. Microglial activation precedes acute neurodegeneration in Sandhoff disease and is suppressed by bone marrow transplantation. *Proc Natl Acad Sci USA.* 2000;97(20):10954–10959.

30. Walkley SU, Suzuki K. Consequences of NPC1 and NPC2 loss of function in mammalian neurons. *Biochim Biophys Acta.* 2004;1685(1–3):48–62.

31. Hong YB, Kim EY, Jung SC. Upregulation of proinflammatory cytokines in the fetal brain of the Gaucher mouse. *J Korean Med Sci.* 2006;21(4): 733–738.

32. Ohmi K, Greenberg DS, Rajavel KS, Ryazantsev S, Li HH, Neufeld EF. Activated microglia in cortex of mouse models of mucopolysaccharidoses I and IIIB. *Proc Natl Acad Sci USA.* 2003;100(4):1902–1907.

33. Simonaro CM, D'Angelo M, He X, Eliyahu E, Shtraizent N, Haskins ME, Schuchman EH. Mechanism of glycosaminoglycan-mediated bone and joint disease: implications for the mucopolysaccharidoses and other connective tissue diseases. *Am J Pathol.* 2008;172(1):112–122.

34. Qiao X, Lu JY, Hofmann SL. Gene expression profiling in a mouse model of infantile neuronal ceroid lipofuscinosis reveals upregulation of immediate early genes and mediators of the inflammatory response. *BMC Neurosci.* 2007;8:95.

35. d'Azzo A, Tessitore A, Sano R. Gangliosides as apoptotic signals in ER stress response. *Cell Death Differ.* 2006;13(3):404–414.

36. Pelled D, Lloyd-Evans E, Riebeling C, Jeyakumar M, Platt FM, Futerman AH. Inhibition of calcium uptake via the sarco/endoplasmic reticulum Ca^{2+}-ATPase in a mouse model of Sandhoff disease and prevention by treatment with N-butyldeoxynojirimycin. *J Biol Chem.* 2003;278(32):29496–29501.

37. Pelled D, Trajkovic-Bodennec S, Lloyd-Evans E, Sidransky E, Schiffmann R, Futerman AH. Enhanced calcium release in the acute neuronopathic form of Gaucher disease. *Neurobiol Dis.* 2005;18(1):83–88.

38. Shen JS, Meng XL, Moore DF, Quirk JM, Shayman JA, Schiffmann R, Kaneski CR. Globotriaosylceramide induces oxidative stress and up-regulates cell adhesion molecule expression in Fabry disease endothelial cells. *Mol Genet Metab.* 2008 Nov;95(3):163–168.

39. Wei H, Kim SJ, Zhang Z, Tsai PC, Wisniewski KE, Mukherjee AB. ER and oxidative stresses are common mediators of apoptosis in both neurodegenerative and non-neurodegenerative lysosomal storage disorders and are alleviated by chemical chaperones. *Hum Mol Genet.* 2008;17(4): 469–477.

40. Eskelinen EL, Saftig P. Autophagy: a lysosomal degradation pathway with a central role in health and disease. *Biochim Biophys Acta.* 2009;1793(4): 664–673.

41. Venugopal B, Mesires NT, Kennedy JC, Curcio-Morelli C, Laplante JM, Dice JF, Slaugenhaupt SA. Chaperone-mediated autophagy is defective in mucolipidosis type IV. *J Cell Physiol.* 2009;219(2):344–353.

42. Settembre C, Fraldi A, Jahreiss L, Spampanato C, Venturi C, Medina D, de Pablo R, Tacchetti C, Rubinsztein DC, Ballabio A. A block of autophagy in lysosomal storage disorders. *Hum Mol Genet.* 2008;17(1):119–129.

43. Pacheco CD, Lieberman AP. The pathogenesis of Niemann-Pick type C disease: a role for autophagy? *Expert Rev Mol Med.* 2008;10:e26.

44. Yang Z, Vatta M. Danon disease as a cause of autophagic vacuolar myopathy. *Congenit Heart Dis.* 2007;2(6):404–409.

45. Raben N, Hill V, Shea L, Takikita S, Baum R, Mizushima N, Ralston E, Plotz P. Suppression of autophagy in skeletal muscle uncovers the accumulation of ubiquitinated proteins and their potential role in muscle damage in Pompe disease. *Hum Mol Genet.* 2008;17(24):3897–3908.

46. Nedelsky NB, Todd PK, Taylor JP. Autophagy and the ubiquitin-proteasome system: collaborators in neuroprotection. *Biochim Biophys Acta.* 2008; 1782(12):691–699.

47. Quantock AJ, Meek KM, Fullwood NJ, Zabel RW. Scheie's syndrome: the architecture of corneal collagen and distribution of corneal proteoglycans. *Can J Ophthalmol.* 1993;28(6):266–272.

48. Alroy J, Haskins M, Birk DE. Altered corneal stromal matrix organization is associated with mucopolysaccharidosis I, III and VI. *Exp Eye Res.* 1999; 68(5):523–530.

49. Hinek A, Wilson SE. Impaired elastogenesis in Hurler disease: dermatan sulfate accumulation linked to deficiency in elastin-binding protein and elastic fiber assembly. *Am J Pathol.* 2000;156(3):925–938.

50. Ma X, Tittiger M, Knutsen RH, Kovacs A, Schaller L, Mecham RP, Ponder KP. Upregulation of elastase proteins results in aortic dilatation in mucopolysaccharidosis I mice. *Mol Genet Metab.* 2008;94(3):298–304.

51. Tatano Y, Takeuchi N, Kuwahara J, Sakuraba H, Takahashi T, Takada G, Itoh K. Elastogenesis in cultured dermal fibroblasts from patients with lysosomal beta-galactosidase, protective protein/cathepsin A and neuraminidase-1 deficiencies. *J Med Invest.* 2006;53(1–2):103–112.

52. Hinek A, Pshezhetsky AV, von Itzstein M, Starcher B. Lysosomal sialidase (neuraminidase-1) is targeted to the cell surface in a multiprotein complex that facilitates elastic fiber assembly. *J Biol Chem.* 2006;281(6):3698–3710.

53. Pryor PR, Reimann F, Gribble FM, Luzio JP. Mucolipin-1 is a lysosomal membrane protein required for intracellular lactosylceramide traffic. *Traffic.* 2006;7(10):1388–1398.

54. Soyombo AA, Tjon-Kon-Sang S, Rbaibi Y, Bashllari E, Bisceglia J, Muallem S, Kiselyov K. TRP-ML1 regulates lysosomal pH and acidic lysosomal lipid hydrolytic activity. *J Biol Chem.* 2006;281(11):7294–7301.

55. Griffin LD, Gong W, Verot L, Mellon SH. Niemann-Pick type C disease involves disrupted neurosteroidogenesis and responds to allopregnanolone. *Nat Med.* 2004;10(7):704–711.

56. Liao G, Cheung S, Galeano J, Ji AX, Qin Q, Bi X. Allopregnanolone treatment delays cholesterol accumulation and reduces autophagic/lysosomal dysfunction and inflammation in Npc1-/- mouse brain. *Brain Res.* 2009; 1270:140–151.

57. Fuller M, Brooks DA, Evangelista M, Hein LK, Hopwood JJ, Meikle PJ. Prediction of neuropathology in mucopolysaccharidosis I patients. *Mol Genet Metab.* 2005;84(1):18–24.

58. Randall DR, Colobong KE, Hemmelgarn H, Sinclair GB, Hetty E, Thomas A, Bodamer OA, Volkmar B, Fernhoff PM, Casey R, Chan AK, Mitchell G, Stockler S, Melancon S, Rupar T, Clarke LA. Heparin cofactor II-thrombin complex: a biomarker of MPS disease. *Mol Genet Metab.* 2008;94(4):456–461.

59. Beesley CE, Young FP, Finnegan N, Jackson M, Mills K, Vellodi A, Cleary M, Winchester BG. Discovery of a new biomarker for the mucopolysaccharidoses (MPS), dipeptidyl peptidase IV (DPP-IV; CD26), by SELDI-TOF mass spectrometry. *Mol Genet Metab.* 2009;96(4):218–224.

60. Groener JE, Poorthuis BJ, Kuiper S, Hollak CE, Aerts JM. Plasma glucosylceramide and ceramide in type 1 Gaucher disease patients: correlations with disease severity and response to therapeutic intervention. *Biochim Biophys Acta.* 2008;1781(1–2):72–78.

61. Deegan PB, Cox TM. Clinical evaluation of biomarkers in Gaucher disease. *Acta Paediatr Suppl.* 2005;94(447):47–50.

62. Yoshino M, Watanabe Y, Tokunaga Y, Harada E, Fujii C, Numata S, Harada M, Tajima A, Ida H. Roles of specific cytokines in bone remodeling and hematopoiesis in Gaucher disease. *Pediatr Int.* 2007;49(6):959–965.

63. Aerts JM, Groener JE, Kuiper S, Donker-Koopman WE, Strijland A, Ottenhoff R, van Roomen C, Mirzaian M, Wijburg FA, Linthorst GE, Vedder AC, Rombach SM, Cox-Brinkman J, Somerharju P, Boot RG, Hollak CE, Brady RO, Poorthuis BJ. Elevated globotriaosylsphingosine is a hallmark of Fabry disease. *Proc Natl Acad Sci USA*. 2008;105(8):2812–2817.

64. Vedder AC, Linthorst GE, van Breemen MJ, Groener JE, Bemelman FJ, Strijland A, Mannens MM, Aerts JM, Hollak CE. The Dutch Fabry cohort: diversity of clinical manifestations and Gb3 levels. *J Inherit Metab Dis*. 2007;30(1):68–78.

65. Gupta S, Ries M, Kotsopoulos S, Schiffmann R. The relationship of vascular glycolipid storage to clinical manifestations of Fabry disease: a cross-sectional study of a large cohort of clinically affected heterozygous women. *Medicine (Baltimore)*. 2005;84(5):261–268.

66. Shah JS, Hughes DA, Tayebjee MH, MacFadyen RJ, Mehta AB, Elliott PM. Extracellular matrix turnover and disease severity in Anderson-Fabry disease. *J Inherit Metab Dis*. 2007;30(1):88–95.

67. Vylet'al P, Hůlková H, Zivná M, Berná L, Novák P, Elleder M, Kmoch S. Abnormal expression and processing of uromodulin in Fabry disease reflects tubular cell storage alteration and is reversible by enzyme replacement therapy. *J Inherit Metab Dis*. 2008;31(4):508–517.

68. An Y, Young SP, Kishnani PS, Millington DS, Amalfitano A, Corz D, Chen YT. Glucose tetrasaccharide as a biomarker for monitoring the therapeutic response to enzyme replacement therapy for Pompe disease. *Mol Genet Metab*. 2005;85(4):247–254.

69. Hendriks MM, Smit S, Akkermans WL, Reijmers TH, Eilers PH, Hoefsloot HC, Rubingh CM, de Koster CG, Aerts JM, Smilde AK. How to distinguish healthy from diseased? Classification strategy for mass spectrometry-based clinical proteomics. *Proteomics*. 2007;7(20):3672–3680.

Vignette

In 1968, Elizabeth Neufeld and her colleagues discovered that culturing fibroblast cells lines established from individuals with *MPS-I* (*Hurler syndrome*) together with those obtained from *MPS-II* (*Hunter syndrome*) patients resulted in the clearance of storage material in both cell types. Subsequent studies revealed that the enzyme (α-L-iduronidase), whose deficiency is responsible for *MPS-I*, was synthesized and secreted by the *MPS-II* (iduronate-2-sulfatase deficient) cells, and *vice versa*. Thus, the elimination of storage materials in distinctly affected cell lines could be explained by their ability to capture the 'corrective factor' from the medium.

Stuart Kornfeld and William Sly later discovered that mannose-6-phosphate receptors were involved in the internalization of the secreted enzymes that had the appropriate glycosylation pattern. These studies involved cells obtained from patients with *I-cell disease* (*mucolipidosis II*), in which deficient activity of the enzyme (GlcNac-1-phosphotransferase) precluded the modification of newly synthesized lysosomal enzymes, which resulted in their 'leaking' out of the cell, rather than being directed to the lysosome. The latter phenomenon occurs, as the enzymes are not properly glycosylated, and do not have the 'zip' code to direct their delivery to the lysosome. Thus lysosomal hydrolysis of various substrates does not occur.

These seminal observations became the foundation for bone marrow/cellular transplantation, and also provided the rationale for enzyme replacement therapy as a corrective measure for the *MPS* disorders.

The subsequent availability of animal models for several LSDs enabled investigations to prove that enzyme infusions are safe and can be effective in stabilizing or improving several key features of *MPS*. Currently, regulatory approval has been granted for the use of recombinant enzyme therapy in *MPS-I, II and VI* (*Maroteaux-Lamy syndrome*), based on the outcome of placebo-controlled trials. Although enzyme therapy for the *MPS* disorders has been shown to modify clinical course, its long-term effectiveness needs to be established.

Suggested Reading

Burrow TA, Hopkin RJ, Leslie ND, Tinkle BT, Grabowski GA. Enzyme reconstitution/replacement therapy for lysosomal storage diseases. *Curr Opin Pediatr.* 2007;19(6):628–635.

Clarke LA. The mucopolysaccharidoses: a success of molecular medicine. *Expert Rev Mol Med.* 2008 Jan 18;10:e1.

Pastores GM. Laronidase (Aldurazyme): enzyme replacement therapy for mucopolysaccharidosis type I. *Expert Opin Biol Ther.* 2008;8(7):1003–1009.

6

Current and Emerging Therapies

Unlike other inborn errors of metabolism which involve 'small molecules'* and are treatable by dietary restriction, vitamin supplementation and/or the administration of 'cleansing' drugs (such as carnitine and phenylbutyrate), the management of LSDs relies primarily on therapeutic strategies to reduce or eliminate tissue deposits (Table 6.1).

Current strategies to enhance substrate clearance include either cellular or protein (enzyme) replacement, as a means of restoring intracellular enzyme activity.[1] Alternatively, medications that partially inhibit substrate synthesis may also be administered to reduce the cellular metabolic burden.[2] Therapies under investigation include the use of pharmacologic chaperones, gene therapy and stem cell transplantation.[2]

Increased understanding of the pathogenic role of aberrant inflammation, autophagy and apoptosis may lead to identification of pharmacologic agents that may be used as adjunctive therapies to target these detrimental cellular changes.[3] Supplemental therapies for disease-related problems, such as the use of anti-bone resorbing agents for osteoporosis in patients with *Gaucher disease* have also been considered.[4] In disorders associated with bone and joint problems, as seen in the *MPS* disorders, physical and occupational therapy remain part of a comprehensive approach to patient care.[4]

The main goal of therapy is the preservation of organ function, which can be challenging given the multiplicity of cell types that can be involved in any given LSDs. Furthermore, therapeutic response is likely to be influenced by several disease-related factors, including the presence of

*i.e., defects of amino and organic acid metabolism.

125

Table 6.1.   Therapeutic approaches.

Therapeutic Option	Candidate Diseases
1. Bone marrow transplantation	• Hurler (MPS IH), Maroteaux-Lamy (MPS-VI), globoid-cell leukodystrophy (Krabbe disease), metachromatic leukodystrophy (MLD), α-mannosidosis
2. Enzyme replacement therapy	• Approved for Gaucher disease (GD), Anderson-Fabry disease (AFD), Hurler-Scheie (MPS-I), Hunter (MPS-II) syndrome, Maroteaux-Lamy (MPS-VI), Pompe disease (GSD-II)
3. Substrate reduction therapy	• Approved for GD and Niemann-Pick type C; investigational for AFD, late-onset G_{M2}-gangliosidosis (LOTS)
4. Substrate depletion therapy	• Cystinosis
5. Chaperone-mediated enzyme enhancement	• Proposed but remains investigational for GD and AFD
6. Gene therapy	• Clinical trials conducted in GD (but remains investigational); for other LSD indications pre-clinical trials primarily in mouse models

CNS involvement and extent of pre-existing tissue damage (e.g., fibrosis, necrosis). Thus, disease subtype and clinical stage represent major determinants of outcome. Ultimately, a combination of therapeutic strategies may be necessary to achieve the best results. As with other complex diseases, management of affected individuals requires a multidisciplinary team. In cases where expectations of a treatment response are high, one must be realistic in counseling and sympathetic in the delivery of care to affected individuals and their families.

Cellular Transplantation

The rationale for both cellular and enzyme replacement therapy is metabolic cross-correction; the phenomenon first observed in mixed cell cultures, wherein enzymes secreted by healthy donor cells were internalized and subsequently directed to the lysosomes of deficient cells.[5] The presence of receptors on the surface of cells, specifically mannose-6-phosphate (M6P) receptors, enabled the capture of the secreted or infused enzyme.[5] In this regard, β-glucosidase is exceptional, as the recombinant formulation is routed through the α-mannose receptor, whereas the endogenous enzyme gets to the lysosome via LIMP-2.[6,7]

Cellular replacement is achieved primarily through allogeneic hematopoietic bone marrow/stem cell transplantation (HSCT).[8] The use of neural stem cells (NSC) implanted directly into the brain is under investigation for at least one disorder (*late-infantile neuronal ceroid lipofuscinosis*).[9] Within the CNS, there must be proper integration of donor cells, and differentiation into appropriate cell types. As specialized cell types within the nervous system elaborate neurotransmitters and are involved in conduction of electrical impulses, functional integrity is critical.

Increasingly, donor material is isolated from umbilical cord blood (UCB), cells that are deemed to have greater potential for trans-differentiation, and thus, may have greater facility for tissue-specific regeneration or repair.[8] Additionally, the incidence of graft *versus* host disease appears to be lower following the use of UCB cells, potentially resulting in decreased transplant morbidity. Currently, the high procedure-related morbidity and mortality risks associated with HSCT have limited its general application, primarily to disease subtypes associated with neurodegenerative features.

HSCT is a consideration primarily for disorders associated with primary CNS involvement (e.g., *Krabbe disease*, *Hurler syndrome*, *α-mannosidosis*). Monocytes in the donor pool can traverse the blood-brain-barrier (BBB) and differentiate into microglia (which serve as the source of functional enzyme).[8] The replacement of endogenous microglia by donor cells is estimated to take at least 6 to 9 months, during which time pathogenic influences may remain. This may explain the potential limitations of HSCT, particularly in cases where the diagnosis is delayed. In *Krabbe disease*, over 80% of infantile cases subjected to HSCT in the first few weeks of life were found to have gross motor problems after the age of 2 years, often requiring assistance with ambulation.[8]

In *MPS* disorders, problems related to bone disease remain an issue; thus, response to HSCT is partial, and influenced by disease stage at the time of transplant.[10] Unfortunately, most *MPS* children who undergo

HSCT ultimately require major orthopedic surgery for genu valgum, hip dysplasia, kyphoscoliosis, carpal tunnel syndrome and trigger digits. Disease type is also a major consideration; early attempts have shown no clinical benefit following transplant in patients with *Hunter* and *Sanfilippo syndrome (MPS-III)*, the reasons for these observations are not understood, and may be related to *MPS*-type-specific disease mechanisms.[10]

Donor cells used in stem cell transplantation may be effective not only as replacement for defective host cells and the provision of functional enzyme; stem cells may also serve as a source of trophic factors and anti-inflammatory mediators to promote normal cellular survival or proliferation. Moreover, donor cells can also be modified genetically to regulate and boost the production of a specific enzyme, to maximize the benefit of using UCB or other cell types.[11,12] Studies in the mouse models of *MPS-VII* and *metachromatic leukodystrophy (MLD)* show that transplanting transduced-cells overexpressing the cognate enzyme resulted in a better outcome, when compared with the results seen using non-transduced cells.[11,12]

Enzyme Replacement Therapy (ERT)

The therapeutic approach consists of the regular intravenous infusion of a recombinant enzyme generated in Chinese hamster ovary (CHO) cells; exceptions include idursulfase (for *MPS-II*), velaglucerase (*GD*) and agalsidase alfa (*AFD*), which are derived from human cell lines in which the encoding gene has been activated to overexpress the cognate enzyme.[13,14] Also, there is a recombinant form of glucocerebrosidase (*GD*) generated in carrot cells, which is currently in clinical trials.[15]

Diseases for which ERT is available are those caused by a deficiency of soluble hydrolases (Table 6.2). Treatment of affected patients has proven to be effective in reversing or stabilizing several disease manifestations, and also leads to a reduction or delay in the evolution of major complications.[13,14] Tissues of the reticulo-endothelial system, such as cells within the liver and spleen, are sites that are readily accessible and show the most substantial clearance of storage material. On the other hand, ERT does not alter the ultimate prognosis of diseases associated with CNS involvement, likely because of minimal delivery of intravenously infused enzyme across

Table 6.2. Enzyme replacement therapy.

Disease	Therapeutic Responses
Gaucher	• Improved blood counts, reduction of liver and spleen volume, improved bone density at the lumbar spine
Anderson-Fabry	• Partially mitigates neuropathic pain and gastrointestinal discomfort, modifies course of renal disease in mild to moderate CKD*, reduces left ventricular hypertrophy, does not appear to significantly alter incidence of stroke
MPS I, II and VI	• Reduced urinary GAG excretion, reduced liver and spleen volume, improvement in FVC†, increased endurance, based on distance traveled during a timed walk test
Pompe	• Resolution of cardiomyopathy (infantile-onset cases), stabilization or improvement in muscle strength, respiratory improvement

*CKD — chronic kidney disease; †FVC — forced vital capacity

the BBB. To overcome this problem, intraventricular and intrathecal (IT) administration are being examined as alternative methods for drug delivery. In *MPS-I* patients with signs of spinal cord compression, preliminary findings suggest the potential for clinical benefit;[16] however, safety concerns and the practicality of chronic IT therapy remain to be clarified.

Furthermore, pre-existing bone lesions (such as osteonecrosis and bone infarcts) that are encountered in the glycosphingolipidosis (such as *GD*) are not reversed with ERT; although treatment at an early stage in the disease process appears to halt progression, perhaps because reduced substrate storage dampens the inflammatory processes that occur with macrophage activation in this condition.[4] Unfortunately, the skeletal dysplasia seen in the *MPS* disorders is also not significantly altered, perhaps because of limited access to relevant cell types and the fact that these changes represent abnormal bone formation which starts *in utero*.[4,17] However, increased height has been observed in some children with *MPS* whose therapy was started prior to puberty.[17]

The extent to which ERT will be effective in leading to event-free survival that approximates normal lifespan remains to be established. In adult males with *AFD*, treatment in a proportion of patients has not halted progression of renal and cardiac disease.[18,19] It has been argued that this may be related to the advanced stage of disease prior to initiation of treatment, or the possibility that antibodies against the infused enzyme have an adverse influence on therapeutic response.[18,20]

Antibodies against the infused enzyme have developed in varying proportions of treated patients, but appear to have the least impact among *GD* patients on ERT.[20,21] Several studies have shown that some of the circulating antibodies may inhibit the activity of infused enzyme and/or alter its tissue distribution. In patients with *Pompe disease*, antibody formation in CRIM-negative patients may be a major factor in the poor outcome seen in some of the infantile-onset cases on recombinant enzyme.[22] Studies in *MPS-I* dogs indicate that inducing immune tolerance and the administration of a higher enzyme dose enable greater clearance of tissue deposits;[23] this approach may be considered in patients at risk for developing antibodies, although it would complicate their overall management. More recently, it has been suggested that certain LSDs may be associated with problems in the recycling of the M6P receptor or the internal transit of the infused enzyme towards the lysosome.

Infusion-related reactions, such as fever and rigors, have been reported in ERT-treated patients, although these problems can be readily mitigated in most by a slower rate of enzyme infusion and the administration of appropriate pre-medications.[13] Rare cases of an anaphylactoid reaction have been described, necessitating close monitoring of infused patients, particularly those with *MPS* and *Pompe disease* who may be compromised by pre-existing cardio-pulmonary problems.

Substrate Reduction Therapy (SRT)

The approach involves the use of a drug which inhibits substrate synthesis, so that ultimately the substrate load is within the capacity of the mutant enzyme.[24,25] This approach can potentially have a broader indication than ERT (which is disease-specific), when the drug has action in limiting the concentration of a precursor for several substrates. Ultimately, the clearance of accumulated substrate is dependent on the presence of residual endogenous enzyme activity; thus, this option may be more suitable for patients with mutations associated with the expression of a defective enzyme showing residual activity.

The imino sugar miglustat has been shown to lead to partial gly-cosphingolipid synthesis inhibition and modification of disease course in treated patients with *GD*.[26] As miglustat can reach the CNS and inhibit the formation of G_{M2}-gangliosides, its potential use was explored in patients with late-onset *Tay-Sachs disease* (*LOTS*), *GD type III* and *NPC*.[27–29] In patients with *NPC*, miglustat has been shown to lead to improvement in saccadic eye movements and swallowing,[29] although impact on survival and eventual neurologic prognosis was limited. Unfortunately, the miglustat trials in patients with *LOTS* and *GD type III* failed to show any measurable benefit, perhaps because of the advanced stage of disease suffered by the subjects prior to study enrollment.[27,28]

A more potent agent, GENZ112638 (a P4-ceramide analogue which is currently in clinical trials in *GD* patients), has also shown promising results,[30] although minimal CNS delivery restricts its use to non-neuronopathic disease subtypes.

Diarrhea and weight loss were observed in patients on miglustat, caused by inhibition of the digestion of certain sugars and the associated increase in osmotic load within the intestinal tract.[31] These problems are transient, and their incidence and severity appear to be diminished with careful attention to diet and continued use of the drug. Paresthesias and tremor have also been observed in some patients, necessitating vigilant monitoring of miglustat-treated patients.[31]

For the *MPS* disorders, a significant proportion of the various clinical subtypes is associated with primary CNS involvement, which is not likely to be altered by intravenously administered ERT. The isoflavone genistein has been demonstrated to decrease GAG synthesis in cultured fibroblasts obtained from *MPS* patients, by inhibiting the tyrosine-specific protein kinase activity of the EGF receptor; as a small molecule it may have good CNS penetration.[32] Thus, genistein may be potentially useful for a subset of patients, although its safety and efficacy in the treatment of patients with *MPS* remains to be established.

Substrate Depletion or Modulation Therapy

The oral administration of an aminothiol cysteamine promotes the lowering of cystine content in lysosomes of patients with *cystinosis*, resulting in maintenance of renal function and improved growth.[33] Cysteamine promotes an intralysosomal disulfide interchange which leads to the formation of free cysteine and a conjugated form of cysteine,[33] which is able to leave the lysosome via other transporters. As an eyedrop, cysteamine helps to dissolve the corneal crystals that can develop in these individuals.

Allopregnanolone (ALLO) has been shown to reduce filipin-labeled unesterified cholesterol accumulation in neuronal endosomes/lysosomes in several regions of the brain of the *NPC1* mouse model. Improved myelination was also observed, independent of cholesterol accumulation, a phenomenon possibly related to changes in cell adhesion function. ALLO treatment was also associated with changes in the ratio of LC3-II/LC3-I and levels of cathepsin B and D, indicative of improvement in lysosomal function and the regulation of autophagy. These observations are prompting trials in human patients *with NPC1*.[34]

Chaperone-Mediated Enzyme Enhancement Therapy

The use of pharmacologic chaperones is based on pre-clinical studies that have demonstrated the ability of these agents to enhance residual activity of the mutant enzyme, by preventing its premature degradation within the endoplasmic reticulum (Figure 6.1).[35,36] The effectiveness of this strategy in substantially clearing tissue deposits, and its clinical efficacy in modifying disease phenotype when used as a singular approach remains to be established. The drugs currently in clinical trials include isofogamine for *GD* and the imino sugar *N*-deoxygalactonojirimycin (DGJ) in *AFD*.[37,38] *In vitro* experiments involving cultured cells isolated from affected individuals indicate that both isofogamine and DGJ enhance the residual activity of β-glucosidase and α-galactosidase A (AGAL), respectively.[37,38] As these drugs are also inhibitors of enzyme activity, determination of the appropriate dose and frequency of administration will be critical, to insure enzyme enhancement has the upper hand. Additionally, the intracellular level of enzyme activity that will need to be achieved to ensure complete substrate clearance and prevent its re-accumulation in each of the target disorders is not certain at this point. It is likely that response to pharmacologic chaperones will be dependent on the underlying mutation, and severely deleterious mutations (e.g., leading to inactivation of the catalytic site) are not going to be responsive to this approach. Further studies in animal models and patients with different gene defects are required.

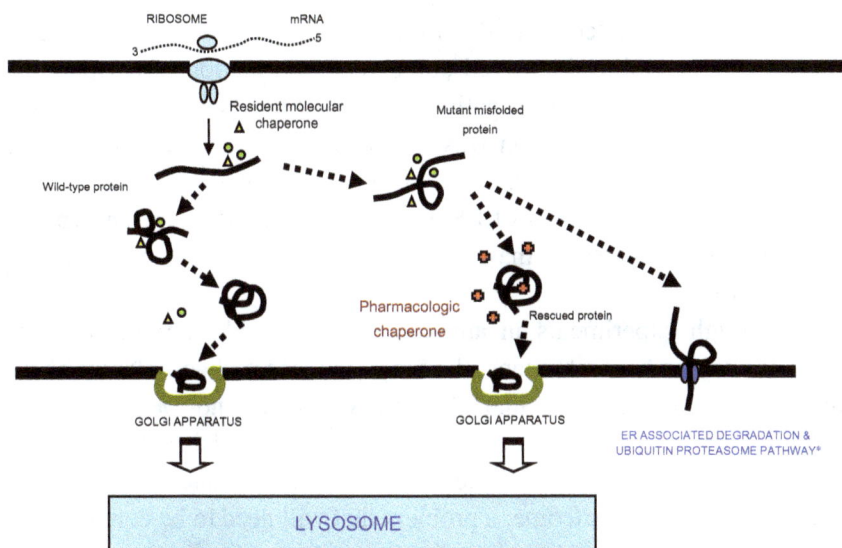

Figure 6.1. Schematic illustration of the mechanism of drug action for pharmacologic chaperones.

*The ubiquitin-proteasome system is involved in the non-lysosomal degradation of intracellular proteins.

A recent study has shown that co-incubation of *Pompe disease* fibroblasts with myozyme (recombinant human α-glucosidase) and miglustat (which acts as a pharmacologic chaperone in this instance) improved correction of the enzyme activity.[39] The findings were attributed to improved myozyme delivery to lysosomes and increased enzyme stability in the presence of miglustat. A similar phenomenon was observed in studies of *AFD* fibroblasts treated with recombinant AGAL and DGJ.[39] These results demonstrate synergy between pharmacological chaperones and ERT.

By preventing the aggregation of mutant misfolded enzyme in the ER, the use of pharmacologic chaperone may also exert action by lowering the unfolded protein responses and ER-stress-related reactions.

Gene Therapy

Apart from correction of the intrinsic enzyme deficiency in transduced cells, gene therapy for LSDs may also lead to secretion of the functional enzyme from these 'corrected' cells which can be taken up by 'uncorrected' cells, enabling improved outcome. Transduction of peripherally mobilized CD34$^+$ cells from patients with *GD* has been performed, but sustained enzyme expression was not seen in these early trials (which involved a retroviral vector).[40] Several other trials have been conducted, primarily in mouse models of LSDs.[41,42] These studies have shown that organ-specific expression may be greater following the use of selected AAV-vectors.

Although experiments in animal models provide a foundation for translational studies in humans, the increased size and complexity of the human brain present particular challenges that may not be clarified by studies in the mouse. Thus, studies in large animal models are preferred.[43] Additionally, immunological rejection of the vector and viral products may lead to adverse outcome, a problem that will need to be contained, to reduce procedure-related risks and promote long-term gene expression. Furthermore, the CNS and synovial joints are sites that can be challenging to treat with systemic gene therapy, and may require direct approaches for delivery of the relevant gene.

In one trial, slowing of disease progression, based on a clinical rating scale and brain imaging, was deemed to have occurred in 10 children with *LINCL* administered AAV2-hCLN2 to 12 sites in the cortex.[44] Serious adverse events, including seizures in one patient who died, were observed; but none of these could be definitively linked to the vector-mediated gene transfer. These preliminary observations are encouraging, but additional studies are clearly required. A major issue for LSDs with CNS pathology, such as *LINCL*, is the diffuse nature of brain involvement. In this condition, the use of transduced neuronal stem cells may be contemplated, but invasive studies involving minors present ethical dilemmas that will require further discussions.

Palliative Care

Symptomatic care remains a mainstay of a comprehensive approach to the management of patients with an LSD, particularly those with major neurologic and skeletal disease. Problems that can interfere with the quality of life of an affected individual include seizures, altered sleep-wake cycles and behavioral problems (such as hyperactivity and aggression).[45–47] Attention to these concerns may reduce the level of frustration expressed by patients and family members, apart from improving the lives of affected individuals.

In *Anderson-Fabry disease*, analgesics and often opiate-type medications are given for acroparesthesia.[48] The frequency and severity of the pain episodes may also be reduced or eliminated by chronic low dose diphenylhydantoin (Dilantin) or carbamazepine (Tegretol) treatment.[48] Additionally, patients are given low dose aspirin or anti-platelet aggregating agents for stroke-prophylaxis and angiotensin converting enzyme inhibitors (e.g., enalapril) for renal protection in those with proteinuria.[48] Dialysis or kidney transplantation is introduced following renal failure, and patients may require a pacemaker or defibrillator for cardiac conduction abnormalities or arrhythmias. Patients with severe heart valve problems may need a mechanical or tissue heart valve replacement, and cardiac transplantation has been performed in patients with cardiomyopathy and heart failure.

Patients with *MPS* who experience sleep apnea benefit from CPAP or BiPAP.[45–47] In *Pompe disease*, pulmonary problems related to weak intercostal and diaphragmatic muscles may necessitate the use of volume ventilators.[49]

Prevention of contractures, which may develop in *MPS* and other LSDs associated with neuromuscular involvement, is important.[4] Physical therapy should include daily stretching, correction of positioning, use of appropriate splints or orthotic intervention, and the provision of adequate support in all positions.[4] In patients with *late-onset Pompe disease* (*acid maltase myopathy*), a high-protein and low-carbohydrate diet and exercise therapy has been reported to slow the deterioration of muscle function (as measured by the Walton scale).[50]

Organ Transplantation

Renal and/or cardiac transplantation have been performed in patients with *AFD*.[51,52] Several patients with *GD* have undergone liver transplantation; in almost all these cases liver failure was due to inter-current problems (e.g., hepatitis B infection).[53] Obviously, these procedures only address problems related to primary organ failure and not the systemic disease burden. Thus, *AFD* patients remain at risk for cerebrovascular disease and other problems that may be ameliorated by ERT. Similarly, post-liver transplant *GD* patients continue to be treated with ERT, to attend to the extrahepatic problems encountered in this condition.

Adjunctive Therapies

As studies in animal models implicate aberrant inflammatory processes in the development of neurodegeneration, it is possible immuno-modulation and other therapies aimed at dealing with downstream disease events may have a positive influence on clinical course. With delineation of relevant disease mechanism, other approaches may come to light.

Recently, it has been suggested that modulation of the calcium concentration in the ER may be one approach to promote proper folding of certain mutant proteins, thereby preventing its premature degradation and facilitating enzyme delivery to the lysosome. Two small calcium channel blockers diltiazem and verapamil were recently shown to restore enzyme function in fibroblasts from patients with *GD*, *α-mannosidosis* and *MPS-IIIB*.[54] The enzyme enhancement may have resulted from induction and up-regulation of a subset of molecular chaperones, including BiP and Hsp40.

Two proteostasis regulators, celastrol and MG-132, have been demonstrated to improve the folding capacity of affected cells from patients with *GD* and *TSD*, by activating the UPR, which mediates the partial restoration of folding, trafficking and function of the cognate enzyme.[55] Thus, the proteostasis regulators may act synergistically with pharmacologic chaperones to enhance residual enzyme activity.

Further Points to Consider

Development of directed therapies for the LSDs was made possible through the Orphan Drug Act, legislation which reduced the manufacturer's overall cost related to the process of seeking regulatory approval, coupled with marketing exclusivity for a defined period, to ensure a return in capital investment made by the pharmaceutical industry and their backers.[13] As commercially available drugs were priced according to 'what the market will bear', the venture has turned out to be hugely profitable for a limited number of biotechnology companies, partly because of the required commitment for chronic, potentially life-long therapy. Ultimately, the value of these novel therapies will be determined, likely in relation to their potential for improving quality of life and promoting event-free survival. Given the multi-systemic nature of most LSDs, combination therapy may ultimately be necessary to achieve an optimal therapeutic outcome, but such an approach has not been formally examined, as yet.

The cost of healthcare delivery for the LSDs is not trivial. Focusing on the care of individual patients to maximize therapeutic outcome revolves around the following: selection of the appropriate patients to treat and the time to initiate therapy; appropriate monitoring to establish rate of disease progression and response to therapy; incorporating changes in drug regimens to achieve an optimal result while taking costs of care into consideration.

It is anticipated that the knowledge gained regarding putative disease mechanisms will translate into development of new therapeutic strategies. In this regard, issues that will need to be addressed include: the feasibility of having a control group in investigations of rare disorders; analysis of therapeutic outcome in patient cohorts with wide heterogeneity in genotypes and clinical expression; the mechanics of getting patients to the few centers with the requisite expertise; and the enrollment of minors in clinical trials, particularly when the therapy or procedures involved are invasive and may lead to pain or discomfort. Thus far, significant inroads have been made in the management of patients with diseases that in the past could only be dealt with in a palliative manner. Building upon this foundation, more gains can be anticipated.

References

1. Platt FM, Lachmann RH. Treating lysosomal storage disorders: current practice and future prospects. *Biochim Biophys Acta*. 2009;1793(4):737–745.
2. Grabowski GA. Treatment perspectives for the lysosomal storage diseases. *Expert Opin Emerg Drugs*. 2008;13(1):197–211.
3. Ballabio A, Gieselmann V. Lysosomal disorders: from storage to cellular damage. *Biochim Biophys Acta*. 2009;1793(4):684–696.

4. Pastores GM. Musculoskeletal complications encountered in the lysosomal storage disorders. *Best Pract Res Clin Rheumatol.* 2008;22(5):937–947.

5. Pastores GM, Barnett NL, Current and emerging therapies for the lysosomal storage disorders. *Expert Opin Emerg Drugs.* 2005;10(4):891–902.

6. Grabowski GA. Delivery of lysosomal enzymes for therapeutic use: glucocerebrosidase as an example. *Expert Opin Drug Deliv.* 2006;3(6):771–782.

7. Reczek D, Schwake M, Schröder J, Hughes H, Blanz J, Jin X, Brondyk W, Van Patten S, Edmunds T, Saftig P. LIMP-2 is a receptor for lysosomal mannose-6-phosphate-independent targeting of beta-glucocerebrosidase. *Cell.* 2007;131(4):770–783.

8. Prasad VK, Kurtzberg J. Emerging trends in transplantation of inherited metabolic diseases. *Bone Marrow Transplant.* 2008;41(2):99–108.

9. Pierret C, Morrison JA, Kirk MD. Treatment of lysosomal storage disorders: focus on the neuronal ceroid-lipofuscinoses. *Acta Neurobiol Exp (Wars).* 2008;68(3):429–442.

10. Prasad VK, Mendizabal A, Parikh SH, Szabolcs P, Driscoll TA, Page K, Lakshminarayanan S, Allison J, Wood S, Semmel D, Escolar ML, Martin PL, Carter S, Kurtzberg J. Unrelated donor umbilical cord blood transplantation for inherited metabolic disorders in 159 pediatric patients from a single center: influence of cellular composition of the graft on transplantation outcomes. *Blood.* 2008;112(7):2979–2989.

11. Sakurai K, Iizuka S, Shen JS, Meng XL, Mori T, Umezawa A, Ohashi T, Eto Y. Brain transplantation of genetically modified bone marrow stromal cells corrects CNS pathology and cognitive function in MPS VII mice. *Gene Ther.* 2004;11(19):1475–1481.

12. Cartier N, Aubourg P. Hematopoietic stem cell gene therapy in Hurler syndrome, globoid cell leukodystrophy, metachromatic leukodystrophy and X-adrenoleukodystrophy. *Curr Opin Mol Ther.* 2008;10(5):471–478.

13. Pastores GM. Enzyme therapy for the lysosomal storage disorders: principles, patents, practice and prospects. *Expert Opin Ther Patents.* 2003;13(8):1157–1172.

14. Burrow TA, Hopkin RJ, Leslie ND, Tinkle BT, Grabowski GA. Enzyme reconstitution/replacement therapy for lysosomal storage diseases. *Curr Opin Pediatr.* 2007;19(6):628–635.

15. Shaaltiel Y, Bartfeld D, Hashmueli S, Baum G, Brill-Almon E, Galili G, Dym O, Boldin-Adamsky SA, Silman I, Sussman JL, Futerman AH, Aviezer

D. Production of glucocerebrosidase with terminal mannose glycans for enzyme replacement therapy of Gaucher's disease using a plant cell system. *Plant Biotechnol J.* 2007;5(5):579–590.

16. Dickson P, McEntee M, Vogler C, Le S, Levy B, Peinovich M, Hanson S, Passage M, Kakkis E. Intrathecal enzyme replacement therapy: successful treatment of brain disease via the cerebrospinal fluid. *Mol Genet Metab.* 2007;91(1):61–68.

17. Clarke LA, Wraith JE, Beck M, Kolodny EH, Pastores GM, Muenzer J, Rapoport DM, Berger KI, Sidman M, Kakkis ED, Cox GF. Long-term efficacy and safety of laronidase in the treatment of mucopolysaccharidosis I. *Pediatrics.* 2009;123(1):229–240.

18. Schiffmann R, Warnock DG, Banikazemi M, Bultas J, Linthorst GE, Packman S, Sorensen SA, Wilcox WR, Desnick RJ. Fabry disease: progression of nephropathy, and prevalence of cardiac and cerebrovascular events before enzyme replacement therapy. *Nephrol Dial Transplant.* 2009;24(7):2102–2111.

19. Banikazemi M, Bultas J, Waldek S, Wilcox WR, Whitley CB, McDonald M, Finkel R, Packman S, Bichet DG, Warnock DG, Desnick RJ; Fabry disease clinical trial study group. Agalsidase-beta therapy for advanced Fabry disease: a randomized trial. *Ann Intern Med.* 2007;146(2):77–86.

20. Linthorst GE, Hollak CE, Donker-Koopman WE, Strijland A, Aerts JM. Enzyme therapy for Fabry disease: neutralizing antibodies toward agalsidase alpha and beta. *Kidney Int.* 2004;66(4):1589–1595.

21. Starzyk K, Richards S, Yee J, Smith SE, Kingma W. The long-term international safety experience of imiglucerase therapy for Gaucher disease. *Mol Genet Metab.* 2007;90(2):157–163.

22. Nicolino M, Byrne B, Wraith JE, Leslie N, Mandel H, Freyer DR, Arnold GL, Pivnick EK, Ottinger CJ, Robinson PH, Loo JC, Smitka M, Jardine P, Tatò L, Chabrol B, McCandless S, Kimura S, Mehta L, Bali D, Skrinar A, Morgan C, Rangachari L, Corzo D, Kishnani PS. Clinical outcomes after long-term treatment with alglucosidase alfa in infants and children with advanced Pompe disease. *Genet Med.* 2009;11(3):210–219.

23. Dickson P, Peinovich M, McEntee M, Lester T, Le S, Krieger A, Manuel H, Jabagat C, Passage M, Kakkis ED. Immune tolerance improves the efficacy of enzyme replacement therapy in canine mucopolysaccharidosis I. *J Clin Invest.* 2008;118(8):2868–2876.

24. Pastores GM, Barnett NL. Substrate reduction therapy: miglustat as a remedy for symptomatic patients with Gaucher disease type 1. *Expert Opin Investig Drugs.* 2003;12(2):273–281.
25. Platt FM, Jeyakumar M. Substrate reduction therapy. *Acta Paediatr Suppl.* 2008;97(457):88–93.
26. Pastores GM. Miglustat: substrate reduction therapy for lysosomal storage disorders associated with primary central nervous system involvement. *Recent Pat CNS Drug Discov.* 2006;1(1):77–82.
27. Shapiro BE, Pastores GM, Gianutsos J, Luzy C, Kolodny EH. Miglustat in late-onset Tay-Sachs disease: a 12-month, randomized, controlled clinical study with 24 months of extended treatment. *Genet Med.* 2009;11(6):425–433.
28. Schiffmann R, Fitzgibbon EJ, Harris C, DeVile C, Davies EH, Abel L, van Schaik IN, Benko W, Timmons M, Ries M, Vellodi A. Randomized, controlled trial of miglustat in Gaucher's disease type 3. *Ann Neurol.* 2008; 64(5):514–522.
29. Patterson MC, Vecchio D, Prady H, Abel L, Wraith JE. Miglustat for treatment of Niemann-Pick C disease: a randomised controlled study. *Lancet Neurol.* 2007;6(9):765–772.
30. McEachern KA, Fung J, Komarnitsky S, Siegel CS, Chuang WL, Hutto E, Shayman JA, Grabowski GA, Aerts JM, Cheng SH, Copeland DP, Marshall J. A specific and potent inhibitor of glucosylceramide synthase for substrate inhibition therapy of Gaucher disease. *Mol Genet Metab.* 2007;91(3):259–267.
31. Pastores GM, Giraldo P, Chérin P, Mehta A. Goal-oriented therapy with miglustat in Gaucher disease. *Curr Med Res Opin.* 2009;25(1):23–37.
32. Jakóbkiewicz-Banecka J, Piotrowska E, Narajczyk M, Barańska S, Wegrzyn G. Genistein-mediated inhibition of glycosaminoglycan synthesis, which corrects storage in cells of patients suffering from mucopolysaccharidoses, acts by influencing an epidermal growth factor-dependent pathway. *J Biomed Sci.* 2009;16:26.
33. Kleta R, Gahl WA. Pharmacological treatment of nephropathic cystinosis with cysteamine. *Expert Opin Pharmacother.* 2004;5(11):2255–2262.
34. Liao G, Cheung S, Galeano J, Ji AX, Qin Q, Bi X. Allopregnanolone treatment delays cholesterol accumulation and reduces autophagic/lysosomal dysfunction and inflammation in Npc1-/- mouse brain. *Brain Res.* 2009;1270:140–151.

35. Pastores GM, Sathe S. A chaperone-mediated approach to enzyme enhancement as a therapeutic option for the lysosomal storage disorders. *Drugs R D*. 2006;7(6):339–348.
36. Fan JQ. A counterintuitive approach to treat enzyme deficiencies: use of enzyme inhibitors for restoring mutant enzyme activity. *Biol Chem*. 2008;389(1):1–11.
37. Steet R, Chung S, Lee WS, Pine CW, Do H, Kornfeld S. Selective action of the iminosugar isofagomine, a pharmacological chaperone for mutant forms of acid-beta-glucosidase. *Biochem Pharmacol*. 2007;73(9):1376–1383.
38. Sugawara K, Tajima Y, Kawashima I, Tsukimura T, Saito S, Ohno K, Iwamoto K, Kobayashi T, Itoh K, Sakuraba H. Molecular interaction of imino sugars with human alpha-galactosidase: insight into the mechanism of complex formation and pharmacological chaperone action in Fabry disease. *Mol Genet Metab*. 2009;96(4):233–238.
39. Porto C, Cardone M, Fontana F, Rossi B, Tuzzi MR, Tarallo A, Barone MV, Andria G, Parenti G. The pharmacological chaperone N-butyldeoxynojirimycin enhances enzyme replacement therapy in Pompe disease fibroblasts. *Mol Ther*. 2009;17(6):964–971.
40. Nimgaonkar MT, Bahnson AB, Boggs SS, Ball ED, Barranger JA. Transduction of mobilized peripheral blood CD34+ cells with the glucocerebrosidase cDNA. *Gene Ther*. 1994;1(3):201–207.
41. Hodges BL, Cheng SH. Cell and gene-based therapies for the lysosomal storage diseases. *Curr Gene Ther*. 2006;6(2):227–241.
42. Sands MS, Haskins ME. CNS-directed gene therapy for lysosomal storage diseases. *Acta Paediatr Suppl*. 2008;97(457):22–27.
43. Haskins M. Gene therapy for lysosomal storage diseases (LSDs) in large animal models. *ILAR J*. 2009;50(2):112–121.
44. Worgall S, Sondhi D, Hackett NR, Kosofsky B, Kekatpure MV, Neyzi N, Dyke JP, Ballon D, Heier L, Greenwald BM, Christos P, Mazumdar M, Souweidane MM, Kaplitt MG, Crystal RG. Treatment of late infantile neuronal ceroid lipofuscinosis by CNS administration of a serotype 2 adeno-associated virus expressing CLN2 cDNA. *Hum Gene Ther*. 2008;19(5):463–474.
45. Muenzer J, Wraith JE, Clarke LA. International consensus panel on management and treatment of mucopolysaccharidosis I. Mucopolysaccharidosis I: management and treatment guidelines. *Pediatrics*. 2009;123(1):19–29.

46. Martin R, Beck M, Eng C, Giugliani R, Harmatz P, Muñoz V, Muenzer J. Recognition and diagnosis of mucopolysaccharidosis II (Hunter syndrome). *Pediatrics*. 2008;121(2):e377–386.

47. Valstar MJ, Ruijter GJ, van Diggelen OP, Poorthuis BJ, Wijburg FA. Sanfilippo syndrome: a mini-review. *J Inherit Metab Dis*. 2008 Apr 4.

48. Eng CM, Germain DP, Banikazemi M, Warnock DG, Wanner C, Hopkin RJ, Bultas J, Lee P, Sims K, Brodie SE, Pastores GM, Strotmann JM, Wilcox WR. Fabry disease: guidelines for the evaluation and management of multi-organ system involvement. *Genet Med*. 2006;8(9):539–548.

49. Kishnani PS, Steiner RD, Bali D, Berger K, Byrne BJ, Case LE, Crowley JF, Downs S, Howell RR, Kravitz RM, Mackey J, Marsden D, Martins AM, Millington DS, Nicolino M, O'Grady G, Patterson MC, Rapoport DM, Slonim A, Spencer CT, Tifft CJ, Watson MS. Pompe disease diagnosis and management guideline. *Genet Med*. 2006;8(5):267–288.

50. Slonim AE, Bulone L, Goldberg T, Minikes J, Slonim E, Galanko J, Martiniuk F. Modification of the natural history of adult-onset acid maltase deficiency by nutrition and exercise therapy. *Muscle Nerve*. 2007;35(1):70–77.

51. Cybulla M, Walter KN, Schwarting A, Divito R, Feriozzi S, Sunder-Plassmann G. On behalf of the European FOS Investigators Group. Kidney transplantation in patients with Fabry disease. *Transpl Int*. 2009;22(4):475–481.

52. Karras A, De Lentdecker P, Delahousse M, Debauchez M, Tricot L, Pastural M, Bruneval P, Zemoura L, Van Huyen DJ, Lidove O. Combined heart and kidney transplantation in a patient with Fabry disease in the enzyme replacement therapy era. *Am J Transplant*. 2008;8(6):1345–1348.

53. Taddei T, Mistry P, Schilsky ML. Inherited metabolic disease of the liver. *Curr Opin Gastroenterol*. 2008;24(3):278–286.

54. Mu TW, Fowler DM, Kelly JW. Partial restoration of mutant enzyme homeostasis in three distinct lysosomal storage disease cell lines by altering calcium homeostasis. *PLoS Biol*. 2008;6(2):e26.

55. Mu TW, Ong DS, Wang YS, Yates JR 3rd, Segatori L, Kelly JW. Chemical and biological approaches synergize to ameliorate protein-folding diseases. *Cell*. 2008;134(5):769–781.

7

Future Prospects

The lysosomal storage disorders (LSD) are inborn errors of compartmentalized metabolism, wherein the deficiency of an enzyme, co-factor or transport protein results in a disruption of lysosomal function. As a consequence, there is accumulation of primary and secondary substrates within several tissues, and initiation of a complex cascade of pathological changes, the full extent of which remains to be delineated. It is likely that several genetic and epigenetic factors influence disease expression, although the identity of these elements has not been clarified at this point.

In closing, I would like to highlight recent reports that are projected to disclose unmarked avenues of investigation, which hopefully will draw in a new generation of researchers into the field. As will be evident in some of the studies described below, several lessons drawn from inquiry into monogenic disorders such as LSDs are leading to fresh insights about other more common human diseases. Section heading are given to anchor discussion, although it is recognized that the various topics covered overlap each other.

Lysosomal Biogenesis and Function

Most studies to elucidate the disease process associated with LSDs have focused on the corollary of interfering with a particular metabolic pathway. The development of novel techniques for examining cellular phenotype is providing new insights into the more global aspects of lysosomal dysfunction. Recently, most lysosomal genes have been shown to exhibit coordinated transcriptional behavior and regulation by the transcription factor EB (TFEB).[1] Under aberrant storage conditions, TFEB translocate from the cytoplasm to the nucleus, resulting in the activation of its target genes. In cultured cells, TFEB overexpression induce lysosomal biogenesis and increase the degradation of complex molecules, such as glycosaminoglycans and huntingtin (the protein which when defective causes Huntington's disease). These findings indicate that a genetic program controls lysosomal biogenesis and function; a search for means to manipulate this program may disclose novel ways to enhance cellular clearance of substrate deposits associated with LSDs and other neurodegenerative diseases.

Pathogenesis

There is a growing recognition that childhood-onset neurodegenerative LSDs may share pathogenic processes in common with those seen in neurodegenerative diseases (e.g., Alzheimer disease and Parkinson disease) that are commonly encountered in the elderly. For instance, in the mouse model of *MPS-IIIB* (*Sanfilippo syndrome type B*), neurons in the medial entorhinal cortex (MEC) have been shown to accumulate several substances, including P-tau (hyperphosphorylated tau).[2] Previously, P-tau buildup has only been described in one other LSD, *Niemann-Pick disease type C* (see Chapter 5). Whole genome microarray analysis to examine differential gene expression in MEC neurons (isolated by laser capture microdissection) in the *MPS-IIIB* mouse revealed increased expression (6- to 7-fold) of *Lyzs*, which encodes lysozyme (reported to induce the formation of P-tau in cultured neurons). In older *MPS-IIIB* mice, P-tau was also seen in the dentate gyrus, an area important for memory. Electron microscopy of dentate gyrus neurons showed cytoplasmic inclusions of paired helical filaments, P-tau aggregates characteristic of tauopathies — a group of age-related dementias that include Alzheimer disease. These observations complement earlier reports of increased intracellular β-amyloid peptide seen in the brain of patients with *MPS-I* and *III*, suggesting convergent pathways of disease.

It has been hypothesized that cells affected with an LSD have increased energy expenditure for biosynthesis due to deficiencies of raw materials sequestered within the lysosome.[3] The resultant energy imbalance could be the basis of decreased adiposity, which has been described in patients with certain LSDs and animal models thereof. Moreover, the negative energy balance, as a result of nutrient deprivation, might induce autophagy, a phenomenon now recognized to be implicated in various LSDs (Chapter 5). Prior studies on LSDs have concentrated on dissecting the nature of the accumulating substrates and downstream consequences. In recent experiments involving the *MPS-I* mouse, metabolite analysis identified deficiencies in simple sugars, nucleotides, and lipids in the livers.[4] In contrast, most amino acids, amino acid derivatives, dipeptides, and urea were elevated, suggesting increased protein catabolism (possibly mediated by increased autophagy). Although it is not certain which of these observations represent compensatory or adaptive changes (as opposed to the consequence of deleterious events), such studies may uncover potential biomarkers that can be used in monitoring disease state. Furthermore, a fuller understanding of intermediary metabolism in the LSDs may unravel pathways that can serve as targets for manipulation to optimize therapeutic outcome. Along these lines, it has been suggested that a secondary benefit of substrate reduction therapy may be the restoration of cellular homeostasis by reducing the demand for raw materials necessary for the *de novo* synthesis of the stored substrates.

Animal Models

Several spontaneously-occurring models have been described in large animals, such as dog, cat and sheep, and many knock-out mouse models have been developed. Studies involving these animal models of LSDs have enabled knowledge of phenotypic expression and putative mechanism(s) of disease. Pre-clinical trials have also helped establish 'proof of principle' for current and emerging therapies.

Of interest are the descriptions of specie-specific differences in clinical presentation, and the apparent influence of background strain on phenotype in studies involving the mouse model. In certain cases, the outcome may reflect differences in metabolic pathways, as shown with sialidase activity in the mouse when compared to humans with β-hexosamindase deficiency (*Tay-Sachs disease*).[5] In most of the cases, the basis for the phenotypic difference is not known, and investigations along these lines may lead to the identification of potential genetic modifiers of disease expression.

As most patients with an LSD are diagnosed after the onset of symptoms, studies involving animal models of disease have been especially valuable in elucidating early features of pathogenesis. In a recent report, a progressive breakdown of axons and synapses in the brains of two different mouse models of *neuronal ceroid lipofuscinosis* (*NCL*) has been described.[6] In the *infantile* and *variant late-infantile NCL* models, synaptic pathology was evident in the thalamus and cortex of the affected mice. Quantitative comparisons of expression levels for a subset of proteins previously implicated in regulation of axonal and synaptic vulnerability revealed changes in proteins involved with synaptic function/stability and cell cycle regulation. These changes were present at pre-/early-symptomatic stages, occurring in advance of morphologically detectable synaptic or axonal pathology. Regional selectivity was also observed, with protein expression changes occurring first within the thalamus and only later in the cortex. There were significant differences in individual protein expression profiles between the two *NCL* models studied; however 2/15 proteins examined (specifically, VDAC1 and Pttg1) displayed significant changes in both models, and may be potentially useful as *in vivo* biomarkers of pre-/early-symptomatic axonal and synaptic vulnerability in the *NCLs*. Such studies may provide insight into the optimal timing of therapeutic intervention to maximize prospects for a good outcome.

Phenotype

The LSDs are often multi-systemic disorders, although a characteristic feature may lead to consideration of a particular diagnosis. In the *MPS* disorders, short stature is a manifestation shared by various subtypes. The cause of shortened long bones is not known. In a series of experiments involving *MPS-VII* mice, chondroitin-4-sulfate (C4S) accumulation in the growth plate was shown to reduce expression of leukemia inhibitory factor (LIF) and STAT3-tyrosine phosphorylation, which resulted in reduced chondrocyte proliferation and ultimately shortened bones.[7] Studies involving animal model of the other *MPS* disorders will be necessary to elucidate whether the same pathways are compromised, as a consequence of storage of distinct glycosaminoglycans (GAG).

Diagnosis

Diagnosis of an LSD can be challenging, particularly in atypical cases where clinical phenotype may overlap with other genetically distinct disorders. In addition, LSDs may result from mutations in genes not currently implicated in disease. A recent study has described the use of comparative proteomics approaches as a means of elucidating the cause of disease in suspected but undiagnosed cases.[8] As most LSDs arise from mutations in genes encoding lysosomal proteins that contain mannose 6-phosphate (M6P), the investigators purified proteins with M6P (by affinity chromatography) from brain autopsy specimens obtained from 23 patients with either confirmed or possible lysosomal disorder. The rationale was that proteins that are decreased or absent in patients compared with controls could represent candidates for the primary defect, and could direct further biochemical or genetics studies. The relative abundance of individual proteins in the mixture was estimated by spectral counting of peptides detected by tandem mass spectrometry. This approach proved to be instrumental in the identification or validation of mutations in two lysosomal proteins, CLN5 and sulfamidase, in the adult form of *NCL*. Application of this technique may lead to identification of factors relevant in initiating or promoting the disease process. Meanwhile, different methods for rapid, cost-efficient multiplex diagnosis continue to be examined.[9]

Blood-Brain Barrier

There is limited characterization of the status of the blood-brain barrier (BBB) in neuronopathic LSDs. It is possible the function of the BBB may be compromised and be an added factor in neuropathology.[10] Furthermore, the BBB may limit the access of various therapies to brain cells; with respect to enzyme replacement therapy, the limited expression of mannose and M6P receptors in the BBB of adults may be a critical issue.[10] Studies in the *MPS-IIIA* mice suggest that M6P receptors may be developmentally regulated,[11] underscoring the need for early therapy.

Modification of the recombinant protein may be required to enhance tissue uptake within sequestered sites, such as the bone and brain. In experiments using human β-glucuronidase (GUS) which has been tagged with an acidic oligopeptide, a more prolonged blood clearance was observed (when compared with the untagged enzyme) and storage was reduced in cortical neurons, hippocampus, and glia cells of affected *MPS-VII* mice.[12] These observations extend earlier findings by the same investigators, involving human GUS whose carbohydrate-dependent receptor-mediated uptake had been inactivated by chemical modification.[13]

More direct approaches for delivering the recombinant enzymes to sites within the brain are also the subject of several on-going studies. These include convection-enhanced delivery and intratechal or intraventricular enzyme administration.[14,15]

Strategies to Improve Therapeutic Outcome

The long-term implications of circulating antibodies that develop against the infused recombinant enzyme in a proportion of treated patients remain to be delineated. There are indications that antibodies inhibit enzyme uptake and can adversely influence outcome.[16,17] These concerns have served as the impetus to examine the potential of modulating immune response to enhance treatment effects. Strategies that have been examined include the use of immunosuppression, and hematopoietic stem cell gene transfer.[18–20] The associated risk–benefit ratio of such approaches will need to be determined, prior to its incorporation in routine clinical practice.

Given the modest responses seen in patients with LSDs who have been treated with M6P receptor-mediated recombinant proteins, and the inherent limitations of this modality with gaining access to certain sites of substrate storage, recent attention has focused on small molecular agents. Interests have also been fostered by recognition of protein folding defects as arising from mutations of the cognate enzyme, and the potential pathologic contributions resulting from activation of endoplasmic reticulum (ER)-stress response (e.g., release of pro-inflammatory cytokines). Different competitive inhibitors are in development as candidate pharmacologic chaperones for various LSDs. These studies have resulted in re-examination of the intracellular factors that influence protein stability, and may offer the possibility of selecting or designing agents that interact with sites remote from the active site or dimmer interface.[21] Alternatively, agents that can enhance the folding of mutant proteins within the ER which have been stabilized by pharmacologic chaperones may be a complimentary approach to consider.[22] The action of pharmacologic chaperones in stabilizing the enzyme may also be used to advantage, when given in conjunction with enzyme replacement therapy.[23]

As an alternative approach to reducing substrate synthesis by means of chemical inhibitors, a biologic option, based on a small interfering RNA procedure to control expression of particular genes, has been proposed. In a set of experiments, aimed at reducing the mRNA levels of four genes (XYLT1, XYLT2, GALTI and GALTII), the efficiency of GAG production in fibroblasts from *MPS-IIIA* patients was considerably reduced.[24]

It is hoped that these studies will result in expansion of the treatment armamentarium, and the introduction of therapies, particularly for LSDs that currently can only be dealt with in a palliative manner. Obviously, further pre-clinical studies are warranted.

References

1. Sardiello M, Palmieri M, di Ronza A, Medina DL, Valenza M, Gennarino VA, Di Malta C, Donaudy F, Embrione V, Polishchuk RS, Banfi S, Parenti G, Cattaneo E, Ballabio A. A gene network regulating lysosomal biogenesis and function. *Science.* 2009;325(5939):473–477.
2. Ohmi K, Kudo LC, Ryazantsev S, Zhao HZ, Karsten SL, Neufeld EF. Sanfilippo syndrome type B, a lysosomal storage disease, is also a tauopathy. *Proc Natl Acad Sci USA.* 2009;106(20):8332–8337.
3. Woloszynek JC, Coleman T, Semenkovich CF, Sands MS. Lysosomal dysfunction results in altered energy balance. *J Biol Chem.* 2007;282(49): 35765–35771.

4. Woloszynek JC, Kovacs A, Ohlemiller KK, Roberts M, Sands MS. Metabolic adaptations to interrupted glycosaminoglycan recycling. *J Biol Chem.* 2009 Aug 21.
5. Sango K, Yamanaka S, Hoffmann A, Okuda Y, Grinberg A, Westphal H, McDonald MP, Crawley JN, Sandhoff K, Suzuki K, Proia RL. Mouse models of Tay-Sachs and Sandhoff diseases differ in neurologic phenotype and ganglioside metabolism. *Nat Genet.* 1995;11(2):170–176.
6. Kielar C, Wishart TM, Palmer A, Dihanich S, Wong AM, Macauley SL, Chan CH, Sands MS, Pearce DA, Cooper JD, Gillingwater TH. Molecular correlates of axonal and synaptic pathology in mouse models of Batten disease. *Hum Mol Genet.* 2009 Jul 29.
7. Metcalf JA, Zhang Y, Hilton MJ, Long F, Ponder KP. Mechanism of shortened bones in mucopolysaccharidosis VII. *Mol Genet Metab.* 2009; 97(3):202–211.
8. Sleat DE, Ding L, Wang S, Zhao C, Wang Y, Xin W, Zheng H, Moore DF, Sims KB, Lobel P. Mass spectrometry-based protein profiling to determine the cause of lysosomal storage diseases of unknown etiology. *Mol Cell Proteomics.* 2009;8(7):1708–1718.
9. la Marca G, Casetta B, Malvagia S, Guerrini R, Zammarchi E. New strategy for the screening of lysosomal storage disorders: the use of the online trapping-and-cleanup liquid chromatography/mass spectrometry. *Anal Chem.* 2009 Jun 25.
10. Begley DJ, Pontikis CC, Scarpa M. Lysosomal storage diseases and the blood-brain barrier. *Curr Pharm Des.* 2008;14(16):1566–1580.
11. Urayama A, Grubb JH, Sly WS, Banks WA. Mannose 6-phosphate receptor-mediated transport of sulfamidase across the blood-brain barrier in the newborn mouse. *Mol Ther.* 2008;16(7):1261–1266.
12. Montaño AM, Oikawa H, Tomatsu S, Nishioka T, Vogler C, Gutierrez MA, Oguma T, Tan Y, Grubb JH, Dung VC, Ohashi A, Miyamoto K, Orii T, Yoneda Y, Sly WS. Acidic amino acid tag enhances response to enzyme replacement in mucopolysaccharidosis type VII mice. *Mol Genet Metab.* 2008;94(2):178–189.
13. Grubb JH, Vogler C, Levy B, Galvin N, Tan Y, Sly WS. Chemically modified beta-glucuronidase crosses blood-brain barrier and clears neuronal

storage in murine mucopolysaccharidosis VII. *Proc Natl Acad Sci USA.* 2008;105(7):2616–2621.

14. Lonser RR, Schiffman R, Robison RA, Butman JA, Quezado Z, Walker ML, Morrison PF, Walbridge S, Murray GJ, Park DM, Brady RO, Oldfield EH. Image-guided, direct convective delivery of glucocerebrosidase for neurono-pathic Gaucher disease. *Neurology.* 2007;68(4):254–261.

15. Dickson P, McEntee M, Vogler C, Le S, Levy B, Peinovich M, Hanson S, Passage M, Kakkis E. Intrathecal enzyme replacement therapy: successful treatment of brain disease via the cerebrospinal fluid. *Mol Genet Metab.* 2007;91(1):61–68.

16. Ponder KP. Immune response hinders therapy for lysosomal storage diseases. *J Clin Invest.* 2008;118(8):2686–2689.

17. Hollak CE, Linthorst GE. Immune response to enzyme replacement therapy in Fabry disease: impact on clinical outcome? *Mol Genet Metab.* 2009;96(1):1–3.

18. Dickson P, Peinovich M, McEntee M, Lester T, Le S, Krieger A, Manuel H, Jabagat C, Passage M, Kakkis ED. Immune tolerance improves the efficacy of enzyme replacement therapy in canine mucopolysaccharidosis I. *J Clin Invest.* 2008;118(8):2868–2876.

19. Joseph A, Munroe K, Housman M, Garman R, Richards S. Immune tolerance induction to enzyme-replacement therapy by co-administration of short-term, low-dose methotrexate in a murine Pompe disease model. *Clin Exp Immunol.* 2008;152(1):138–146.

20. Douillard-Guilloux G, Richard E, Batista L, Caillaud C. Partial phenotypic correction and immune tolerance induction to enzyme replacement therapy after hematopoietic stem cell gene transfer of alpha-glucosidase in Pompe disease. *J Gene Med.* 2009;11(4):279–287.

21. Lieberman RL, D'aquino JA, Ringe D, Petsko GA. Effects of pH and iminosugar pharmacological chaperones on lysosomal glycosidase structure and stability. *Biochemistry.* 2009;48(22):4816–4827.

22. Mu TW, Ong DS, Wang YJ, Balch WE, Yates JR 3rd, Segatori L, Kelly JW. Chemical and biological approaches synergize to ameliorate protein-folding diseases. *Cell.* 2008;134(5):769–781.

23. Benjamin ER, Flanagan JJ, Schilling A, Chang HH, Agarwal L, Katz E, Wu X, Pine C, Wustman B, Desnick RJ, Lockhart DJ, Valenzano KJ.

The pharmacological chaperone 1-deoxygalactonojirimycin increases alpha-galactosidase. A levels in Fabry patient cell lines. *J Inherit Metab Dis.* 2009;32(3): 424–440.

24. Dziedzic D, Węgrzyn G, Jakóbkiewicz-Banecka J. Impairment of glycosaminoglycan synthesis in mucopolysaccharidosis type IIIA cells by using siRNA: a potential therapeutic approach for Sanfilippo disease. *Eur J Hum Genet.* 2009 Aug 19.

Disease Index

153

General Index

www.ingramcontent.com/pod-product-compliance
Lightning Source LLC
Chambersburg PA
CBHW050629190326
41458CB00008B/2196